The Musculoskeletal System at a Glance

Christopher Bulstrode

MCh, FRCS(Orth)
Clinical Reader in Trauma and Orthopaedics
University of Oxford
Oxford

Catherine Swales

MRCP, PhD
Clinical Lecturer in Rheumatology
Nuffield Orthopaedic Centre
Oxford

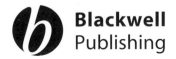

Blackwell
Publishing

Published by Blackwell Publishing Ltd
Blackwell Publishing, Inc., 350 Main Street, Malden, Massachusetts 02148-5020, USA
Blackwell Publishing Ltd, 9600 Garsington Road, Oxford OX4 2DQ, UK
Blackwell Publishing Asia Pty Ltd, 550 Swanston Street, Carlton, Victoria 3053, Australia

First published 2007

1   2007

Library of Congress Cataloging-in-Publication Data

Bulstrode, C. J. K. (Christopher J. K.)
   Musculoskeletal system at a glance / Christopher Bulstrode, Catherine Swales.
      p. ;   cm. – (At a glance series)
   Includes index.
   ISBN-13: 978-1-4051-3515-3 (alk. paper)
   ISBN-10: 1-4051-3515-8 (alk. paper)
   1. Musculoskeletal system.   I. Swales, Catherine.   II. Title.   III. Series: At a glance series (Oxford, England)
   [DNLM: 1. Musculoskeletal System – Handbooks. WE 39 B939m 2006]

   QP301.B8956 2006
   612.7—dc22

                                                                2006014206

A catalogue record for this title is available from the British Library

Set in 9.5/12pt Times by Graphicraft Limited, Hong Kong
Printed and bound in Singapore by COS Printers Pte Ltd

Commissioning Editor: Martin Sugden
Editorial Assistant: Ellie Bonnet
Development Editor: Karen Moore
Production Controller: Debbie Wyer
Artist: Jane Fallows

For further information on Blackwell Publishing, visit our website:
http://www.blackwellpublishing.com

The publisher's policy is to use permanent paper from mills that operate a sustainable forestry policy, and which has been manufactured from pulp processed using acid-free and elementary chlorine-free practices. Furthermore, the publisher ensures that the text paper and cover board used have met acceptable environmental accreditation standards.

Contents

Preface

This book has a broad remit. It is designed to cover everything you need to know as a medical student about the musculo-skeletal system, from fundamentals through to problem solving. Its contents stretch from rheumatology, a multitude of complex medical conditions which challenge the diagnostic skills of the best physicians, through to trauma where big decisions may have to be made very quickly indeed. Within this range, there are a wealth of exciting learning opportunities for medical students. If you are still a little shy with patients and want to build up your confidence and experience, then the rheumatology ward is for you. It has some of the nicest patients in medicine, always happy to see you, to talk, and to show off their cornucopia of physical signs. If you need an adrenaline burst then the trauma room is where you need to go. Lots of excitement and things to do. This book tries to give you the background you need to see and treat patients whose problems are focused around pain, deformity and disability.

The contents of the book are based on the curriculum used by two experienced teachers of medical students who teach rheumatology, trauma and orthopaedics. It focuses on the topics that are essential and important in the course curriculum and which therefore come up in the exams. Enjoy!

Christopher Bulstrode
Catherine Swales
Oxford

Acknowledgements

Guide to anatomical terminology and figures from Chapters 5, 10, 14, 75 and 76 from Faiz, O. & Moffat, D. (2006) *Anatomy at a Glance*, 2nd edn. Blackwell Publishing, Oxford.

Figures from Chapter 22 from Davey, P. (2006) *Medicine at a Glance*, 2nd edn. Blackwell Publishing, Oxford.

Guide to anatomical terminology

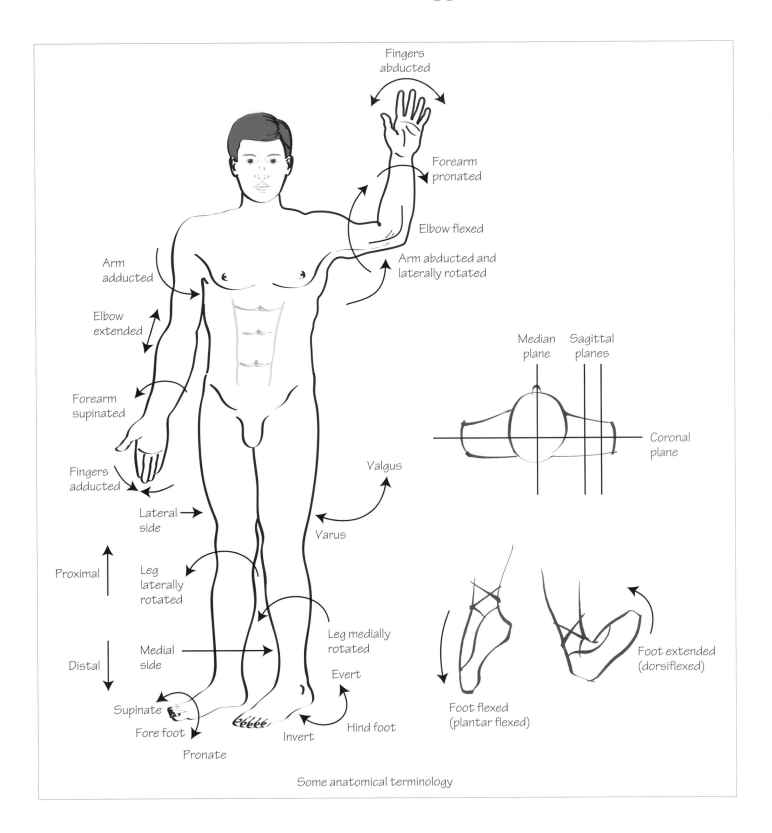

Some anatomical terminology

1 Musculoskeletal structure and function

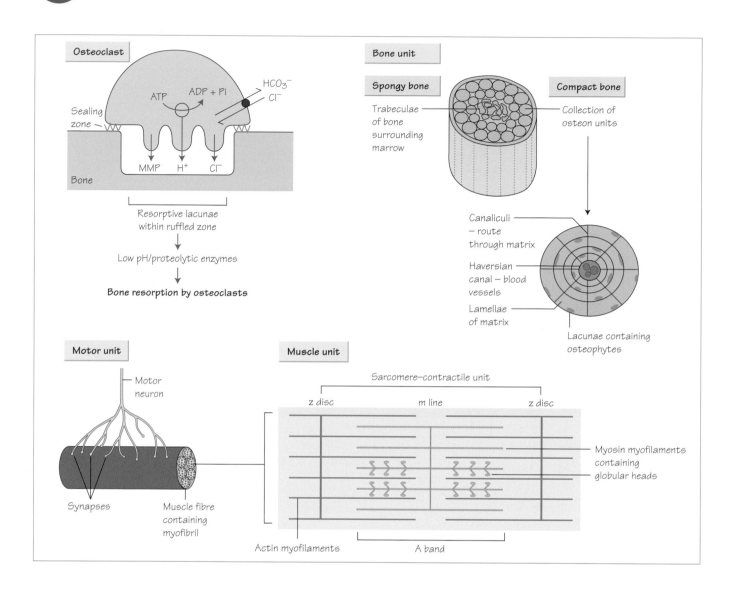

Osteoclast

HCO$_3^-$
Cl$^-$

ATP   ADP + Pi

Sealing zone

Bone

MMP   H$^+$ Cl$^-$

Resorptive lacunae within ruffled zone

Low pH/proteolytic enzymes

Bone resorption by osteoclasts

Bone unit

Spongy bone

Trabeculae of bone surrounding marrow

Compact bone

Collection of osteon units

Canaliculi – route through matrix

Haversian canal – blood vessels

Lamellae of matrix

Lacunae containing osteophytes

Motor unit

Motor neuron

Synapses

Muscle fibre containing myofibril

Muscle unit

Sarcomere–contractile unit

z disc   m line   z disc

Myosin myofilaments containing globular heads

Actin myofilaments   A band

The locomotor system is composed of bone, cartilage, muscle, tendons and ligaments.

Bone

Bone is essentially a mineralised connective tissue. It is composed of cells, a protein matrix and mineral. Three main cell types exist:

1 Osteoblasts ('builders') are responsible for bone formation and lie in sheets on the surface of bone trabeculae.

2 Osteoclasts ('cutters') resorb bone. The plasma membrane adjacent to bone is thrown into folds called the 'ruffled border'; secretion of proteolytic enzymes (e.g. matrix metalloproteinases, MMP) and hydrochloric acid onto the bone surface remove mineral and matrix simultaneously.

3 Osteocytes are mature, relatively inactive osteoblasts that lie in lacunae within bone.

Osteoblasts and osteoclasts are coupled into bone remodelling units that keep adult bone mass relatively constant.

The protein matrix of bone consists largely of type I collagen; the mineral matrix is predominantly hydroxyapatite.

Bone is comprised of two subtypes:

1 Woven bone is formed when bone is laid down rapidly as in the developing fetus, healing fractures or bone-forming tumours.

2 Lamellar bone is laid down slowly. It is structurally strong and forms the adult skeleton. It is arranged in two forms:

- **Compact bone** forms the cortex. It comprises 80% of the skeleton and its contribution is maximal in long bone shafts.
- **Cancellous (spongy) bone** is found in contact with bone marrow cells between the cortices, at the end of long bones and in vertebral bodies.

Cartilage

Articular cartilage is an avascular and aneural shock absorber. It is composed of **chondrocytes**, which create a matrix of **type II collagen**, and **proteoglycans**, which bind water. Adult cartilage consists of four layers – the superficial, middle, deep and calcified zones, which differ in pattern of collagen fibre deposition, and water and cell content.

Muscle

Muscle is formed by fibres that differ according to their twitch rate and fatiguability.

- **Type 1 muscle fibres** are slow twitch (red) fibres that are highly resistant to fatigue. They have abundant mitochondria and are designed to maintain sustained contractions such as needed in posture control.
- **Type 2 muscle fibres** are fast twitch (white) fibres and are designed to produce greater force and rapidity of contraction but fatigue rapidly.

Fibres of similar types group together with a lower motor neuron to form a **motor unit**. Muscle fibres contain **myofibrils** formed by the contractile myofilaments **actin** and **myosin**. The myosin-binding sites on actin are covered by tropomyosin and troponin. However, when an **action potential** reaches a motor unit, stimulation causes calcium release into the surrounding cytoplasm (sarcoplasm). The calcium binds with troponin sites on tropomyosin, revealing the active binding sites and disinhibiting actin filaments. These cross-link with the globular heads on myosin, causing shortening of the motor unit. The muscle relaxes once calcium levels fall and the cross-links are broken.

Tendons and ligaments

Both of these specialised connective tissues are composed of type I collagen. Tendons attach muscle to bone, while ligaments connect bones to one another, supplying support to a joint.

2 Calcium homeostasis and bone metabolism

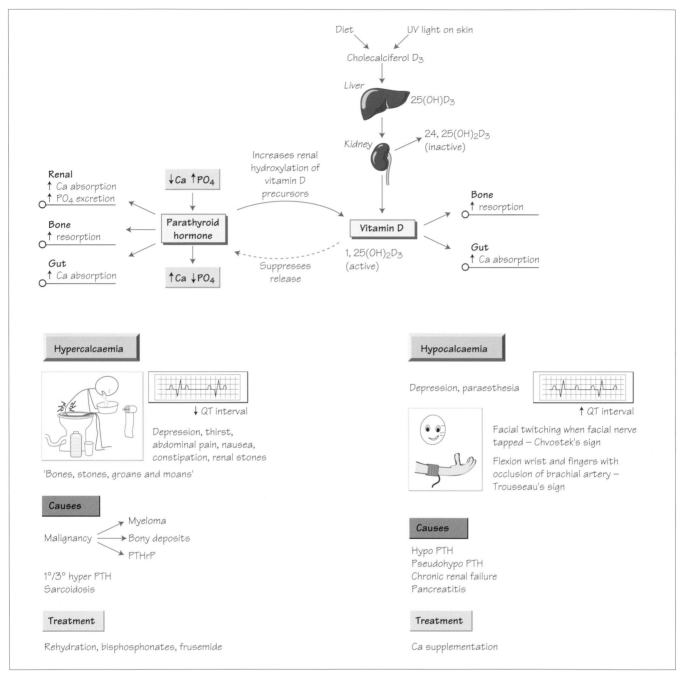

Diet   UV light on skin

Cholecalciferol D₃

Liver

25(OH)D₃

Kidney

24, 25(OH)₂D₃ (inactive)

Increases renal hydroxylation of vitamin D precursors

Renal
↑ Ca absorption
↑ PO₄ excretion

↓Ca ↑PO₄

Parathyroid hormone

Vitamin D

1, 25(OH)₂D₃ (active)

Bone
↑ resorption

Bone
↑ resorption

Gut
↑ Ca absorption

↑Ca ↓PO₄

Suppresses release

Gut
↑ Ca absorption

Hypercalcaemia

↓ QT interval

Depression, thirst, abdominal pain, nausea, constipation, renal stones

'Bones, stones, groans and moans'

Causes

Malignancy → Myeloma
→ Bony deposits
→ PTHrP

1°/3° hyper PTH
Sarcoidosis

Treatment

Rehydration, bisphosphonates, frusemide

Hypocalcaemia

Depression, paraesthesia

↑ QT interval

Facial twitching when facial nerve tapped – Chvostek's sign

Flexion wrist and fingers with occlusion of brachial artery – Trousseau's sign

Causes

Hypo PTH
Pseudohypo PTH
Chronic renal failure
Pancreatitis

Treatment

Ca supplementation

The basics

The skeleton is more than a structural framework. During constant cycles of bone formation and resorption, it plays a vital role in calcium homeostasis. **Calcium** is the most abundant mineral in the body and 99% of it is contained in bone. Half of plasma calcium is bound to albumin and is therefore inactive. Calcium results must be adjusted to account for albumin levels by adding or subtracting 0.02 mmol/l for each g/l by which the albumin is below or above 40 g/l, respectively.

Calcium homeostasis and bone metabolism are principally governed by **vitamin D** and **parathyroid hormone**. Bone meta-bolism is also modulated by calcitonin, glucocorticoids, sex hormones, growth hormone and thyroxine.

Vitamin D

This fat-soluble vitamin is found in the diet and its precursors are also generated in the skin in response to sunlight. Following renal and hepatic hydroxylation, the active component 1,25-dihydroxy-D₃ is released. Its actions are:
- *Gut*: increases calcium absorption from the small bowel.
- *Bone*: increases mineralisation and resorption.

Parathyroid hormone

Parathyroid hormone (PTH) is released in response to low plasma calcium levels. Its overall function is to increase plasma calcium and decrease plasma phosphate levels via actions on the gut, bone and renal tract:

- *Gut*: increases intestinal absorption of calcium.
- *Bone*: increases osteoclastic resorption of bone.
- *Renal*:
   increases calcium reabsorption and phosphate excretion;
   increases renal hydroxylation of vitamin D precursors.

Vitamin D and PTH levels are interlinked: PTH responds to low levels of vitamin D by increasing renal hydroxylation of vitamin D precursors into the active form; high levels of vitamin D feedback to inhibit PTH release.

Disorders of calcium homeostasis
Hypercalcaemia

Elevated calcium levels can cause abdominal pain, nausea, constipation, polyuria, depression and renal stones. They shorten the Q-T interval. The most common cause is malignancy (myeloma, bony metastases, PTH-related protein release from some tumours) or primary hyperparathyroidism. Treatment is with rehydration and frusemide or bisphosphonates.

Hypocalcaemia

The main symptoms of hypocalcaemia are depression and paraesthesia. Obstruction of the brachial artery causes carpopedal spasm (Trousseau's sign) and tapping the facial nerve causes the facial muscles to twitch (Chvostek's sign). The Q-T interval is prolonged. Causes include (pseudo)hypoparathyroidism, chronic renal failure or pancreatitis. Treatment is with calcium supplementation and reversal of the underlying cause.

Hyperparathyroidism
Primary hyperparathyroidism

Inappropriate production of PTH in the presence of a raised calcium level. Most commonly due to a single adenoma but carcinoma and hyperplasia may also be responsible. It causes the symptoms of hypercalcaemia as discussed above and biochemical testing reveals a raised calcium, unsuppressed PTH (i.e. normal or high plasma level), reduced phosphate and elevated alkaline phosphatase. There may be radiological evidence of bone resorption (brown tumours, pepper-pot skull). Treatment is surgical.

Secondary hyperparathyroidism

Appropriate production of PTH in the presence of a low calcium level. The most likely cause is chronic renal failure.

Tertiary hyperparathyroidism

Inappropriate and autonomous production of PTH following prolonged secondary hyperparathyroidism. Calcium is elevated, and treatment is as for primary disease.

Hypoparathyroidism
Primary hypoparathyroidism

Reduced PTH secretion due to autoimmune destruction of the parathyroid glands or their surgical removal. It causes symptoms of hypocalcaemia. Calcium is reduced, phosphate elevated and alkaline phosphatase normal. Treatment is with alfacalcidol.

Pseudohypoparathyroidism

Similar symptoms and treatment to primary condition, but aetiology is due to end-organ resistance to PTH, so hormone levels may rise. Additional features include a round face and short metacarpals/tarsals.

Pseudopseudohypoparathyroidism

Phenotypic appearance of pseudohypoparathyroidism but normal endocrine and biochemical features.

Disorders of bone metabolism
Osteomalacia and rickets

Inadequate mineralisation of osteoid before epiphyseal closure causes rickets, and in the mature skeleton causes osteomalacia. The bone is soft but of normal density, in contrast to osteoporosis. Patients with osteomalacia present with bone pain and fractures. It also induces a waddling gait due to a proximal myopathy.

The commonest causes of osteomalacia are vitamin D deficiency due to:

- poor diet;
- inadequate sun exposure;
- malabsorption;
- renal disease.

Biochemical testing reveals a mildly reduced or normal calcium and phosphate with an elevated alkaline phosphatase. X-rays demonstrate evidence of defective mineralisation and Looser's zones (low density bands of bone extending inwards from the cortex). Treatment is with vitamin D supplementation.

Children with rickets have deformed bones due to bowing and may experience symptoms of hypocalcaemia (see above). Vitamin D-resistant rickets occurs when there is diminished renal hydroxylation of precursors or end-organ resistance to the active form. These patients require large doses of active vitamin D supplementation.

Paget's disease

Paget's disease causes increased bone turnover due to disordered osteoblastic/clastic activity. The resultant bone is enlarged, deformed and weak. The disease is rare under 40 years but increases with age and affects 3% of those over 55 years of age. Although Paget's disease causes enlargement of the skull, femur, clavicle and tibia (which bows forming the characteristic sabre tibia), it is often detected incidentally due to biochemical assessment for other reasons. Complications include bone pain, fractures, compressive neural deafness and, rarely, osteogenic sarcoma and high output cardiac failure. The calcium is normal in the absence of a fracture, but the alkaline phosphatase is dramatically elevated. In addition, urinary hydroxyproline, a marker of bone turnover, is elevated. X-rays reveal osteolytic lesions and sclerosis. Treatment is aimed at bone pain with bisphosphonates, calcitonin or mithramycin.

Taking a history

Introduction	Introduce self – give your name and say who you are Check patient's name Explain what you want to do Check that the patient is comfortable
Patients problems and hopes	Open questions. Explore what is troubling the patient, what they think is wrong and what they are hoping will be done for them
Clarify diagnosis	Closed questions. Try to work out the most likely diagnoses
Systemic enquiry	Questions should be comprehensive but relevant only to fitness for treatment proposed including significant co-morbid conditions, and social issues which may affect recovery and discharge
Closure	Summarise the points. Ask if patient wants any further information

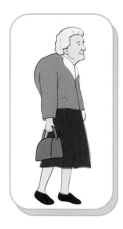

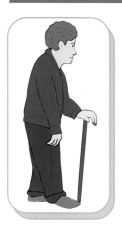

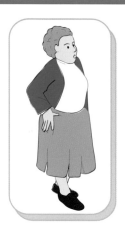

Performing an examination

Introduction	Ask patient to 'Point where it is most tender' Check for other problems/injuries. Wash your hands
Expose	Both limbs. One joint above and below
Use both sides for comparison	
Look	Skin – redness, scars, wounds Soft-tissues – swelling/wasting Bone – deformity
Check neurovascular status	
Feel	Skin – temperature, sensation, sweating Soft-tissues – tenderness, effusion, pulses Bone – tenderness, osteophytes
Move	Active – if necessary demonstrate movement to patient Passive – watch patient's face especially when moving beyond active range Resisted and special tests for stability
Closure	Thank patient, check comfort, check for any questions

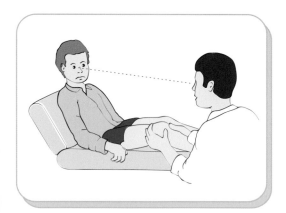

NB ○ The GALS system is an excellent screening tool
   ○ For detailed examination of the hand in rheumatoid arthritis, see Chapter 21 'The rheumatological history'

Determining the underlying aetiology of locomotor disease requires a directed history and examination, but an overall screening system is crucial to ensure that no feature is overlooked. In addition the locomotor history can be employed in the systems review of any general medical or surgical situation.

This chapter will focus on a validated screening tool for the locomotor system, the **GALS locomotor screen** (Doherty *et al.*, 1992, *Annals Rheum. Dis*. 51:1165–9). Detailed and regional history and examination is covered in subsequent chapters.

'GALS (gait, arms, legs, spine)' locomotor screen

Screening questions

If the answer to the following questions is 'No', there is unlikely to be major locomotor pathology.

- 'Have you any pain or stiffness in your muscles, joints or back?'
- 'Can you dress yourself completely without any difficulty?'
- 'Can you walk up and down stairs without any difficulty?'

Screening examination

The examination is broken down into gait, arms, legs and spine, and any abnormality in appearance or movement is documented and a regional, directed history and examination undertaken. It should be performed with the patient in light underwear, allowing close inspection of each area following a few simple commands.

Gait

- Ask the patient to walk a short distance and then turn around:
  Is the gait smooth and symmetrical?
  Normal arm swing, stride length, heel strike, stance and toe-off?
  Able to turn quickly?

Arms

Ask the patient to follow these instructions:
- '*Put your arms behind your head*':
  Assesses the glenohumeral, sternoclavicular and acromioclavicular joints.
- '*Put your arms straight*':
  Tests full elbow extension.
- '*Put your hands in front*':
  Any wrist/finger swelling or deformity?
  Able to extend fingers fully?
- '*Turn your hands over*':
  Tests supination/pronation (superior and inferior radioulnar joints).
  Normal palms? No swelling, wasting or erythema?
- '*Make a fist*':
  Assesses power grip.
- '*Pinch finger to thumb*':
  Assesses precision pinch/dexterity.
- Metacarpal squeeze test:
  Evidence of tenderness/synovitis?

Legs

Inspect whilst standing
- Normal quadriceps bulk/symmetry?
- Knee swelling or deformity?
- Forefoot/midfoot/arches normal?

Examine while lying
- Flex the hip with knee flexed:
  Crepitus? Limitation?
- Passively internally rotate each hip in flexion:
  Pain/restriction?
- Press on patella:
  Patellofemoral tenderness?
  Knee effusion?
- Metatarsal squeeze test:
  Evidence of synovitis?
- Inspect soles for abnormal callosities:
  Evidence of abnormal weight bearing?

Spine

Inspect whilst standing, from behind
- Muscle bulk normal and symmetrical?
- Is the spine straight?

Inspect whilst standing, from the side
- Normal lordosis?
- Evidence of kyphosis?
- '*Bend forward to touch toes*':
  Lumbar spine flexion normal?
- Press over midpoint of supraspinatus:
  Hyperalgesia of fibromyalgia?

Observe from front
- '*Tilt head towards shoulders*'
  Normal lateral neck flexion?

Documentation

Clinical findings can be quickly recorded thus:

G	√	
	Appearance	Movement
A	√	√
L	√	√
S	√	√

A tick denotes a normal finding. If an abnormality is detected, the tick is replaced with a cross and further clinical details are documented under the chart.

'Look, feel, move' system

Combining the GALS screen with the more detailed 'look, feel, move (active, passive and restricted)' system in regional problems will ensure that every patient with locomotor pathology is comprehensively and adequately assessed.

X-ray Request Card

Name	Write tidily
Address	Use sticky labels if possible
Imaging	Don't order views. Describe the side, area, and the diagnosis which needs excluding – put 'Please' at the end
Clinical indications	Give as much useful information as possible Put your name and contact details clearly

The alignment of the femoral neck is all wrong. That leads your eye to the fracture line

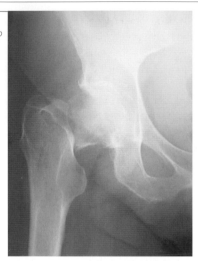

Reading an X-ray

❶ Check Name / Date / Side
❷ Check margins. What is included, what not
❸ Trace skin, soft tissues, fluid levels, looking for swelling or wasting
❹ Trace outlines of bones for alignment and cortical discontinuities. Also check joints for thickness of joint space narrowing, sclerosis, cysts, and osteophytes (OA) or osteopaenia and erosions (RA)
❺ Check inside of bone for lytic lesions and sclerosis
❻ Check other views
❼ Compare with any other (older) films for change over time

X-ray of bone tumour. Note the swelling visible within the soft tissues, as well as the change in the cortical margin

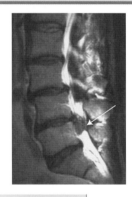

Prolapsed intervertebral disc pressing on nerve roots showing clearly on MRI

CT reconstruction of the lumbar spine showing a crush fracture of a vertebral body

MRI of same tumour confirms extent of tumour in the soft tissues

Modalities of imaging

	Use	Disadvantage
Ultrasound		
Bounces sound off soft tissue interfaces	Dynamic visualisation of soft tissues	Cannot see through bone
Plain X-ray		
Shines X-rays through tissues onto screen	Cheap. Shows bone outline well	Radiation dose. Not good on soft tissues
CT (computerised tomography)		
Reconstructs X-ray beams from many directions	Enhances X-ray image allowing images of slices of tissue to be created improving detail and definition	Radiation dose Expensive
MRI (magnetic resonance imaging)		
Strong magnetic field reverses radio signals emitted by tissues analysed	Shows soft tissues well No radiation	Expensive Claustrophobic

Introduction

A simple system for requesting and reading radiographs should ensure that you do not ever miss abnormalities.

Requesting an X-ray examination

Always fill in your forms tidily; remember there is no harm in adding 'please' to the request form. The radiographer and radiologist need to know where to find the patient and who to send the report to; they must be able to read these details.

When requesting an examination that uses ionising radiation you are responsible for ensuring that the risk is worth the potential clinical benefit. If in doubt ask a radiologist. The radiographer is allowed to perform examinations only when the indications conform with written protocols and standard guidelines; for unusual examinations you will be asked to justify the exposure to a radiologist.

As a general rule do not order specific views. It is the radiographer's job to decide on the views, based on the disease you want to prove or exclude. For example, if you want to exclude slipped upper femoral epiphysis in a child, the radiographer will perform special views to do this. The more information that you give about the history and examination, the better the report you are likely to get back from the radiologist.

Interpreting an X-ray examination

As in all imaging, check the name, side and date. Check to see that there is more than one view and if there are any previous studies. Looking for changes over time is much more sensitive for identifying disease than looking at a single set of images. The following is one system for checking X-rays.

Coverage

First check the margin of the images and decide what structures are included and, more importantly, which are not!

Outlines

Trace the skin outline and make sure this is normal, not swollen. Trace any lines in the soft tissues, looking for fluid levels and evidence of swelling or wasting of structures. Finally trace the edges of the bone margins, looking for steps or breaks in the cortex.

Texture

Check the bones, looking for lytic areas, coarsening of the trabeculae or loss of cortical/medullary differentiation. Finally, check the alignment of the bones and joints taking into account the position the patient was in during the examination.

Review areas

Before you finish, check the parts of the image that are important clinically and look specifically for the diseases that you are worried about. Then review the areas that you have found difficult in the past and those where others commonly make mistakes. Areas behind other structures such as the heart and the very edge of the image are examples, but your experience will create the most useful list.

Asking for help

If you do not know what examination to request or how to interpret the images that you receive, take the problem to a radiologist and ask for help. They are often very shrewd clinicians and are invariably keen to help. Read the written reports and compare them with your findings; this provides a safety net and a learning opportunity.

Pros and cons of the different imaging methods

Plain radiographs

- They are quick and simple to organise.
- They show bones well, but soft tissues are poorly seen.
- They involve radiation and so should be used with caution.

Ultrasound

- Ultrasound is very good at showing soft tissues, and can be used while the patient moves. This can be especially useful in studying sports injuries.
- It does not use ionising radiation and is well tolerated by patients.
- It does, however, require a highly skilled operator.

Computerised tomography (CT)

- This uses the highest doses of ionising radiation routinely encountered in diagnostic imaging but is better at showing soft tissue lesions than plain X-rays.
- It also gives far better three-dimensional visualisation of structures in the body and shows fine details in cross-section.

Magnetic resonance imaging (MRI)

- MRI is very useful at showing soft tissues, especially oedema which may surround infections or tumours.
- However, it cannot obtain a useful signal from healthy bone cortex and fracture lines may be difficult to see.
- It does not involve ionising radiation, and gives good three-dimensional imaging.
- Some patients cannot tolerate the confined space and others cannot be examined for safety reasons (pacemakers, etc.).

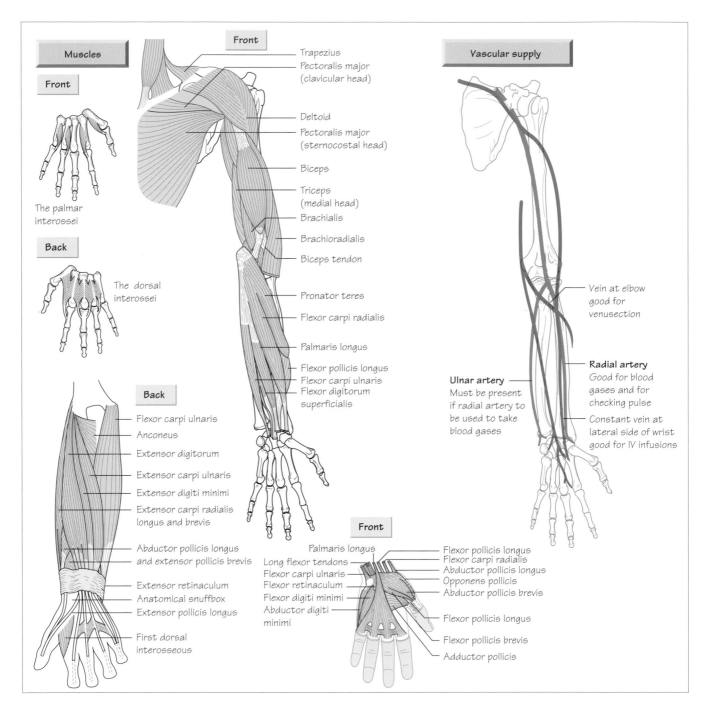

Function

One of the great steps forward in human evolution was the freeing up of the forelimbs for using tools. The human hand is now primarily adapted to hold and manipulate objects. The arms have evolved to enable the hands to be accurately placed, and firmly held, in space in as many positions as possible.

Nerves

The nerve supply to the upper limb arises from the lower cervical and upper thoracic spine (C3 to T3). One of the main nerves to the hand (the **median nerve**) passes into the hand through the narrow carpal tunnel under the flexor retinaculum where it can be compressed (**carpal tunnel syndrome**). The other main nerve to the hand, the **ulnar nerve**, is also at risk for entrapment as it passes through a groove in the bones behind the medial side of the elbow joint. The **digital nerves** to the fingers are very easily injured by any penetrating wound to the hand or fingers.

Vessels

The blood supply of the upper limb passes through the upper arm

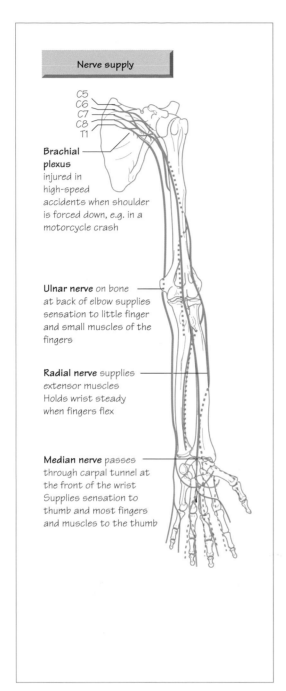

Nerve supply

C5
C6
C7
C8
T1

Brachial plexus injured in high-speed accidents when shoulder is forced down, e.g. in a motorcycle crash

Ulnar nerve on bone at back of elbow supplies sensation to little finger and small muscles of the fingers

Radial nerve supplies extensor muscles Holds wrist steady when fingers flex

Median nerve passes through carpal tunnel at the front of the wrist Supplies sensation to thumb and most fingers and muscles to the thumb

position makes it convenient for taking a pulse and for obtaining blood for arterial gas analysis.

Movement

The shoulder joint moves around on the end of a spoke (the collar bone) with the scapula gliding over the muscles of the chest wall. The shoulder girdle and shoulder joint itself work together to produce a very large range of movement. The shoulder joint itself is a very open cup compared with the hip joint.

Anatomical relationships in relation to pathology

The head of the **humerus** is stabilised and controlled by a ring of muscles that all converge into a single sleeve of tendon enclosing the shoulder joint itself and inserting into the articular margin of the humerus. Part of this rotator cuff must slide under the acromion as it overhangs the joint. It is here that it is susceptible to rubbing, inflammation and pain. It can even tear, as its blood supply and hence capacity for repair is poor (see p. 21).

The radial nerve wraps itself closely around the shaft of the humerus as it winds down from the brachial plexus in the axilla to pass in front of the lateral side of the elbow joint. If the humerus is fractured it is easily damaged.

The elbow joint allows the hand to bend up close to the shoulder or stretch out to the full length of the arm. It also contributes with the wrist joint to the complex manoeuvre of pronation and supination, where the radius and ulna bones fold across each other to allow the hand to rotate along its length. The large muscles controlling both the wrist and fingers arise on either side of the elbow joint, the extensors arising on the lateral side and the flexors from the medial epicondyle.

At the wrist the **radius** has become the dominant bone, spinning around the small ulna head to allow pronation and supination of the hand. The wrist joint is very mobile in all planes giving the hand further mobility. It is stabilised by the balanced contraction of the flexors against the extensor muscles.

The hand

The key to the anatomy of the hand is the **thumb**, which is able to rotate out of the line of the other fingers and oppose the other fingers. This allows the hand to power grip, manipulate a key or pick things up with the tips of the fingers. This dexterity relies on:
• *Sensation* to the finger tips (to feel where things are).
• *Power* in the muscles controlling the fingers and thumb (allowing them to open and then close around an object).
• *Proprioception* (so that the brain knows where the hand is).
• *Mobility* of the joints of the arms (to enable the hand to be put and then held where it is needed).

Opposition of the thumb is controlled by muscles served by the median nerve, so damage to this nerve reduces the key role of the thumb in opposition. The intrinsic muscles of the hand are controlled by the ulnar nerve. These muscles allow the fingers to spread apart and for the fingers to remain straight while they bend at their base, a key requirement for picking things up with the finger tips. Any stiffness in the hand as a result of injury or inflammation or any loss of sensation has a quite disproportionate effect on the function of the hand.

along a single artery so any damage to that artery from external trauma or an embolus will critically compromise the blood supply to the hand. Both nerves and vessels are easily damaged in the upper limb, but cannot be seen on X-ray, so always check distal neurovascular status whenever examining a limb.

In the crease of the elbow (the antecubital fossa) there are large veins (easier to feel than to see), which are excellent for taking blood and for giving fluid in an emergency. At the wrist on the lateral (radial side) there is a large constant vein which is a favourite choice for siting the needle for an intravenous infusion. In the forearm the blood supply passes through a rigid muscle compartment (containing the flexor muscles of the forearm). Swelling in this compartment can produce a **compartment syndrome** (see Chapter 41). The **radial artery** can also be felt easily at the wrist as it passes over the front of the radial head. Its

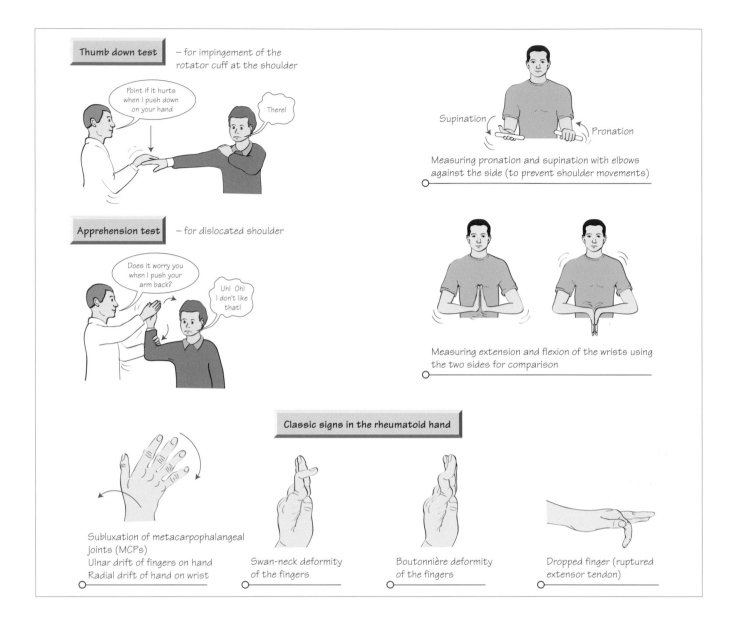

Introduction
Problems in the upper limb may arise from nerve entrapment in the neck, so always check the neck when examining the upper limb. Do not forget to use both sides for comparison and to check distal neurovascular status.

History
• In *trauma* a clear description of how the limb was injured will usually give the likely diagnosis.
• In *chronic problems*, check for early morning pain and stiffness (inflammatory joint disease).

Look
Shoulder
The **acromion** (the point of the shoulder) is much more prominent when the shoulder has dislocated. Even after relocation the acromion may appear prominent again after some weeks as there is usually wasting of the deltoid muscle over the shoulder due to bruising of the circumflex nerve. A prominent lump over the end of the clavicle is the result of injury to the **acromio-clavicular joint** which may sublux and then become arthritic.

Elbow
Hard lumps may form on the back of the elbow (**gouti tophi**), also a favourite site for **psoriasis** (silvery scaly skin on the extensor surface). Any injury to the elbow tends to leave it stiff with loss of flexion and extension.

Wrist
Swelling around the wrist is common in inflammatory joint disease.

Hand and fingers

- Wasting of the base of the thumb occurs if there is damage to the median nerve, especially at the wrist.
- Damage to the ulnar nerve produces wasting in the clefts between the fingers.
- Inflammatory arthritis affects the hands in particular, producing a number of characteristic deformities (see Chapter 22).
- Dupuytren's contracture commonly affects the little and then the ring finger, curling them into the palm (see p. 20).

Feel

The clavicle, acromioclavicular joint and shoulder joint are close to the skin and so are easy to feel. Similarly the bones and joints of the elbow, wrist and hand can all be felt through the skin. Lumps and areas of tenderness can be identified and linked to the underlying anatomical structures.

The ulnar nerve can be felt in the groove between the olecranon and the medial epicondyle at the back of the elbow. If it is tender and sends shock waves down the arm when pressed or tapped, it may be inflamed because it is getting trapped in the groove. Similarly the median nerve may get trapped at the wrist under the flexor retinaculum (**carpal tunnel syndrome**). It also produces a tingling sensation when percussed if it is inflamed (Tinel's sign).

Move

- *Shoulder*. The functional range of the shoulder can be checked by asking the patient to put their hands behind their head, then straight up, straight forward, out to the side and finally bring the hand up the back from below. Use both sides for comparison.
- *Elbow*. If the arms are then held straight forward, flexion and extension of the elbows can be compared by watching the patient from the side.
- *Forearm*. Finally, with the upper arms by the side and the forearms facing straight forward, pronation and supination of the forearm can be checked without the patient being able to use the shoulder to confuse the measurements.
- *Wrist*. Wrist movements can be checked by asking the patient to get into a prayer position then to raise the elbows as far as possible (the exact opposite manoeuvre will check wrist flexion).
- *Finger*. Finger movements can be checked quickly by first asking the patient to make a fist, then unroll the hand to a flat palm and then touch each finger tip to the tip of the thumb in turn. A **trigger finger** can be diagnosed by finding one finger is late in extending and then goes with a jump as the thickened flexor tendon (which can be felt) passes in to the narrow flexor tendon tunnel in the finger.

Resisted movements

- The **thumb down test** is diagnostic of rotator cuff inflammation. The patient should hold the arms out straight with each arm facing 45 degrees forward of straight out sideways. The hand is set so that the thumb is pointing down. If there is a sharp pain in the shoulder when the examiner pushes the hand down against resistance then the test is positive.
- The **apprehension sign** is a feeling of deep unease that patients feel when the shoulder is pushed into extension with the upper arm abducted and the forearm externally rotated. It is strong evidence that the shoulder has been dislocated in the past, and is still unstable.
- Getting the patient to grip your fingers tests the power of both flexors and extensors of the wrist (as the fingers cannot flex properly unless the wrist can be held extended).
- Testing the patient's ability to spread their fingers apart checks the power of the intrinsic muscles of the hand (ulnar nerve).

Special tests

In the case of suspected nerve damage you will need to plot areas of loss of sensation as well as weakness and wasting of individual muscles. Then, by reference to a specialist test, you should be able to work out which nerve(s) are damaged and at which level. Loss of sensation in the hand is best determined using two point discrimination using the other side for comparison.

Carpal tunnel syndrome

Tapping with your finger tip over the front of the patient's wrist (where the median nerve passes under the flexor retinaculum) produces electric shocks running down into the fingers if the median nerve is being compressed (**Tinel's test**). **Phalen's test** involves flexing the patient's wrist while pressing hard on the median nerve at the front of the wrist. After 30 seconds the patient will find their fingers going numb.

Ulnar neuritis

The ulnar nerve frequently gets trapped in the groove on the medial side of the elbow as it passes round the back of the joint. Pressure or tapping on the irritated nerve will produce electric shocks down the arm into the ulnar side of the hand.

Tips

- The best veins at the elbow for taking blood are felt and not seen
- The vein on the lateral side of the wrist is good for siting drips
- Nerves and vessels lie close to bones and joints in the arm and are prone to injury
- Stiffness in the hand produces severe disability
- Always check distal neurovascular status

7 Problems presenting in the arm

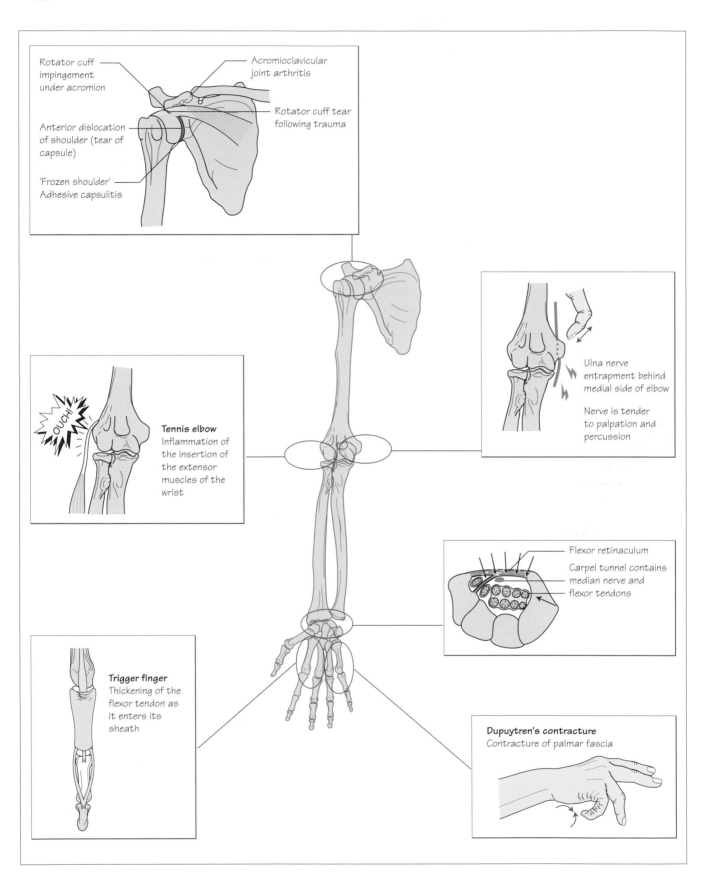

Rotator cuff impingement under acromion

Acromioclavicular joint arthritis

Rotator cuff tear following trauma

Anterior dislocation of shoulder (tear of capsule)

'Frozen shoulder' Adhesive capsulitis

Tennis elbow
Inflammation of the insertion of the extensor muscles of the wrist

OUCH!

Ulna nerve entrapment behind medial side of elbow

Nerve is tender to palpation and percussion

Flexor retinaculum

Carpel tunnel contains median nerve and flexor tendons

Trigger finger
Thickening of the flexor tendon as it enters its sheath

Dupuytren's contracture
Contracture of palmar fascia

Shoulder
Function
Loss of shoulder movement severely compromises the function of the upper limb. A patient with limited mobility in the shoulder should, if possible, be able to put their hand behind the head to brush their hair, behind the back to wipe their bottom, and flex forward to bring their hand to the mouth to eat. Scars on the shoulder can be very disfiguring if they form keloid.

Presentation
• **Rotator cuff impingement.** Several of the muscles around the shoulder insert into a cuff around the head of the humerus, which then inserts into the edge of the glenoid. This rotator cuff has a poor blood supply and must pass through the narrow cleft between the head of the humerus and the acromion. The underside of the acromion becomes beaked with age. It may then rub on the underside of the acromion producing a painful arc. This can produce weakness as well as pain. The acromion can be trimmed back using an arthroscope. Major tears in the rotator cuff can be repaired but unfortunately the blood supply is poor, so healing is not always good.
• **Frozen shoulder.** Strenuous use of the shoulder (such as painting a ceiling) or injury to a shoulder can lead to the gradual onset of a frozen shoulder. Over a period of days and weeks the shoulder becomes stiffer and more painful until the pain dominates the patient's sleeping and waking hours. The natural history of the condition is that over a period of months the pain and stiffness gradually improve until near full function is restored. There appears to be no treatment that can cure the condition or even hasten its natural history.
• **Arthritis of the shoulder (glenohumeral joint)** is common and painful. Fusion of the joint leaves a fairly good range of movement because the scapula is so mobile on the thorax. A shoulder replacement should give pain relief and even better movement, but it will wear out in time.

Arthritis of the acromioclavicular joint
The acromioclavicular joint is commonly injured following a fall onto the point of the shoulder, but the pain from this injury usually settles spontaneously in time. If the joint is then unstable, it may develop arthritis and produce a painful lump on the point of the shoulder. This interferes with rucksack straps. The joint can be excised without loss of function. This should relieve the pain.

Elbow
Function
The movements of the elbow are flexion, extension, and pronation and supination. If **flexion** is lost, the patient may not be able to bring the hand to their mouth. If **extension** is lost, they may not be able to reach things with the hand. **Pronation** and **supination** are crucial in positioning the hand, and loss of this movement significantly reduces the function of the upper limb. Cosmesis is a problem in the elbow if there is a growth abnormality and the elbow is left with a major varus or valgus deformity.

Presentation
• **Ulnar nerve entrapment.** The ulnar nerve can become trapped in the cubital tunnel at the back of the elbow. If this occurs, there may be numbness and wasting on the ulnar one and a half fingers of the hand and wasting of the interosseous muscles. The nerve can be released surgically.
• **Tennis elbow.** A common problem, which produces pain in the elbow whenever the patient grips something, pronates their forearm or fully flexes the wrist. Each of these manoeuvres puts strain on the common extensor tendon origin on the lateral epicondyle of the elbow. A similar problem over the common flexor origin (medial epicondyle) is called **Golfer's elbow**. Physiotherapy or local steroid injection sometimes helps.
• **Arthritis in the elbow** is not uncommon, particularly in rheumatoid arthritis. If it is the radial head that is particularly painful, this can be removed, but elbow replacements are becoming increasingly successful and can produce a painless, strong and mobile elbow joint.

Wrist and hands
Presentation
• **Arthritis in the wrist** commonly follows trauma or inflammatory arthritis. Fusion of the wrist can be useful because it relieves pain, stabilises the joint and improves the strength of grip.
• **Carpal tunnel syndrome.** Most common in middle-aged females and during pregnancy, the patients describe hanging their hand out of bed at night to relieve the pain and numbness. They also notice that they are clumsy, dropping things all the time. On examination there is wasting of the muscles at the base of the thumb, and loss of feeling in the thumb and first two fingers. Nerve conduction studies show the median nerve trapped at the wrist. Steroid injections and splinting may help but surgical decompression of the carpal tunnel will relieve symptoms more reliably.

Dupuytren's contracture
A contracture in the fascia in the palm of the hand draws the fingers into flexion (usually the little and ring finger). The condition runs in families. If caught early the tightening fascia can be removed surgically and function is returned to the hand. If it is left late, amputation of the obstructing fingers may be the only option.

Trigger finger
Repeated trauma to the palm of the hand may lead to thickening of the flexor tendons to the fingers. They may then not be able to run freely in and out of the narrow mouth of the tunnels through which they pass from the palm into the finger. If this happens the finger jams (triggers), flexing with a click, then refusing to extend until helped when once again it triggers. Steroid injection may help. Surgical treatment merely involves opening the mouth of the tendon tunnel slightly.

Tips
• The shoulder frequently gets an impingement problem
• The elbow joint has the ulnar nerve ('funny bone') running close to it
• The median nerve gets trapped at the wrist—carpal tunnel syndrome
• Trigger fingers look normal until the patient tries to move them

---

Injuries to the musculoskeletal system are commonly associated with injuries to nerve and blood supply, so always check distal neurovascular status

Most skeletal injuries are associated with a soft tissue injury—check for it

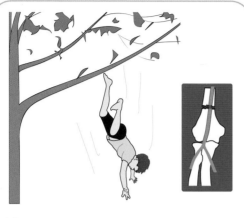

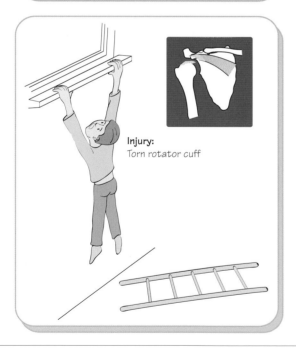

Injury:
Supra-condylar fracture of humerus
Associated injury:
Tear of brachial artery, loss of circulation to lower arm and compartment syndrome

Injury:
Torn rotator cuff

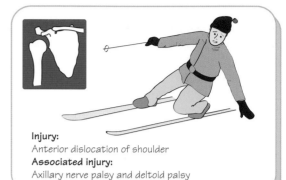

Injury:
Anterior dislocation of shoulder
Associated injury:
Axillary nerve palsy and deltoid palsy

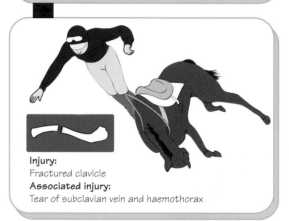

Injury:
Fractured clavicle
Associated injury:
Tear of subclavian vein and haemothorax

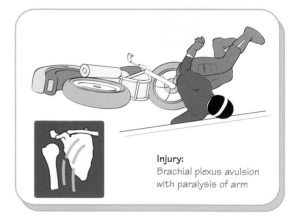

Injury:
Brachial plexus avulsion with paralysis of arm

Introduction

The arm is most commonly injured in a fall when it is used to protect the head and face as well as cushion the fall. Never forget to check ABC (see p. 78), for injuries elsewhere in the body and distal neurovascular status. In high energy accidents (such as falls from a motorcycle) the **brachial plexus** may be torn. This is a devastating injury often leaving a useless arm and very severe causalgia-type pain.

Conversely the **clavicle** is only a thin spoke holding the shoulder complex out and away from the midline. It is therefore easy to break. However, it also heals quickly and has great powers of remodelling if there is a malunion. The joints at each end, especially the **acromioclavicular joint**, can also be subluxed or even dislocated.

Dislocation of the shoulder

The shoulder joint itself allows a large range of movement and as a result is prone to dislocation. This is almost always anterior. The patient has frequently had the problem before and will tell you exactly what the diagnosis is, and even how it can be reduced quickly. Reduction is relatively simple immediately after the injury (the arm just needs to be pulled straight). Later, once muscle spasm has set in, strong analgesia or even an anaesthetic may be needed to get the shoulder back into joint. Treatment is then gentle mobilisation while waiting for the torn tissues around the shoulder joint to heal. If dislocations are repeated, surgery to repair the soft tissues around the shoulder may be needed.

Any patient who has had a dislocation of the shoulder is liable to another. If the arm is put into the position in which the dislocation can occur (above their head and forced backwards) they will become very worried about what might happen next. This is known as an '**apprehension sign**' (see p. 18).

Posterior dislocations are much rarer but are also easy to miss since to the inexperienced eye the anteroposterior radiograph of the shoulder appears normal, and a lateral view may be difficult to obtain. However, the history is very characteristic as posterior dislocations are classically caused by epileptic fits, electric shocks and forced restraint in violent or psychotic patients. Once an index of suspicion is raised by the unusual history, the diagnosis on examination and investigation should be easier to make.

Fractured head of the humerus

This injury is commonest in the elderly who have osteoporosis. If the fragments have lost their blood supply or cannot be reduced to create a useful joint surface, a shoulder joint replacement may be the best treatment. A similar explosive fracture can occur at the lower end of the humerus in the elbow joint. The same treatment principles apply.

Torn rotator cuff

A sudden force on the shoulder, such as a slip from a ladder, may put a large load through the muscles around the shoulder or on their common insertion into the rotator cuff. This will produce weakness in the power of abduction of the arm. In young patients these tears can be repaired surgically. However, in the elderly the poor blood supply and the weakening of the cuff may make a repair impossible to perform, so the patient may have to accept the disability.

Elbow

A fall on the outstretched arm can fracture the bones of the elbow. In children a fall out of a tree or off a swing can produce a **greenstick fracture of the distal radius**. But it can also fracture the **proximal end of the radius** where the bone is driven onto the end of the humerus. The blood in the elbow joint produces a tense painful effusion which can easily be relieved by aspiration and injection of some local anaesthetic. If the radial head is too badly crushed for repair it may need removing and can be replaced with an artificial one.

A more sinister fracture after the same type of fall occurs in the humerus just above the elbow joint. This is a **supracondylar fracture of the humerus**, common in children. The brachial artery lies immediately in front of the bone at this point so this can be damaged by a spike of bone. Bleeding can also track down into the forearm muscles raising the pressure in this compartment. When the fracture is reduced, it is best held in plaster with the elbow flexed up as much as possible. If there is any more bleeding, then either the dressing or the fascia of the forearm muscle itself can produce a **compartment syndrome** (see Chapter 41). The circulation to the hand and the ease with which the fingers can be extended needs to be carefully monitored for at least 12 hours. If there is any suggestion of circulatory compromise, then the plaster must be removed and if that does not lead to a rapid improvement, an urgent fasciotomy will be needed.

Forearm

The **radius** and **ulna** can be broken by a twisting fall. As the two bones work together to produce pronation and supination, it is important to obtain an accurate reduction and fixation if full movement is to return. This is best obtained with open reduction and internal fixation.

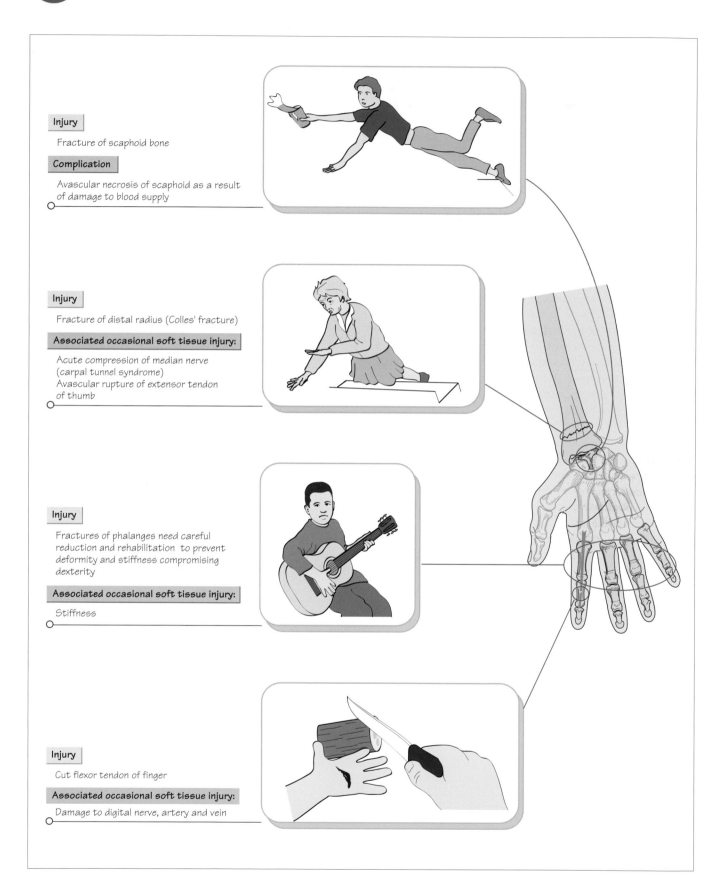

Injury

Fracture of scaphoid bone

Complication

Avascular necrosis of scaphoid as a result of damage to blood supply

Injury

Fracture of distal radius (Colles' fracture)

Associated occasional soft tissue injury:

Acute compression of median nerve (carpal tunnel syndrome)
Avascular rupture of extensor tendon of thumb

Injury

Fractures of phalanges need careful reduction and rehabilitation to prevent deformity and stiffness compromising dexterity

Associated occasional soft tissue injury:

Stiffness

Injury

Cut flexor tendon of finger

Associated occasional soft tissue injury:

Damage to digital nerve, artery and vein

Introduction
Trauma to the hand is common but also important because it can cause cosmetic and functional damage out of all proportion to the severity of the initial injury.

History and examination
Both will be important in determining the structures likely to have been injured. A stabbing injury may damage a nerve, while a crushing injury could lead to a compartment syndrome in the intrinsic muscles. Distal neurovascular status must always be tested as nerve damage is easy to miss.

Falls on the hand
Fractures of the distal radius are very common, especially in the elderly with osteoporosis. The fracture produces a classic 'dinner fork'-type deformity (the Colles' fracture). Because the bones are crushed together, the fracture is stable. So, if it is decided to leave the fracture as it is rather than reduce it, a soft removable splint for comfort may be all that is needed. This will be much easier for the patient to cope with than the heavy plaster that is needed for many weeks if the fracture is reduced and so made unstable.

A distal radial fracture in the non-elderly is a very different injury and should not be called a Colles' fracture. It is a high velocity injury in hard bone where the fracture enters the joint and is unstable. This fracture almost certainly needs open reduction with internal fixation using a moulded plate if stiffness and arthritis in the joint are to be avoided.

Falls may also damage the **carpal bones**. The commonest of these results in tenderness over the base of the thumb, and is the result of a **scaphoid fracture**. The diagnosis is important because a fracture across the waist of this bone may lead to avascular necrosis of the distal pole. Unfortunately the fracture is not always visible on the initial X-rays so treatment may need to be started on the basis of suspicion rather than proof. If the bone is still tender after a week to 10 days of immobilisation, then a further set of X-rays at this time will be much more reliable because if there is a fracture the cleft will now be more open. Even if the scaphoid is not broken the ligaments between the carpal bones can be torn and the bones themselves subluxed or dislocated. The X-rays can be tricky to interpret so if there is severe pain and swelling in the wrist and no obvious fracture, an expert opinion should be sought.

Cuts
Cuts in the hand can easily damage nerves, vessels and tendons. They can also leave **foreign bodies** in the hand that can be difficult to see by eye or on X-ray. The pain, swelling and bleeding can make examination very difficult. Very careful examination is needed to exclude **digital nerve damage**.

If there is any possibility of a retained foreign body or damage to tendons, end vessels or nerves, formal exploration will need to be undertaken with a tourniquet to control bleeding, a regional or general anaesthetic and time to perform any repairs. This will be best performed in an operating theatre, where a clear view can be obtained. Nerves will need repairing under a microscope and tendons will need moving as soon as possible after repair to avoid adhesions. Extensor tendons are much easier to repair than flexor tendons and tend to move better afterwards. Flexor tendons run in fibrous tunnels into the fingers. If a cut tendon is repaired where it runs in these tunnels the join tends to jam in the narrow tunnel and scar tissue forms preventing all movement. Tendon grafts are needed to move the site of the repair out of the danger zones and into the palm where mobilisation is possible.

Fractures of the metacarpals and phalanges
Metacarpal head fractures caused by punching can usually be left unreduced as they are stable and cause no functional problem. However, **spiral phalangeal fractures** need careful reduction and holding. The fracture is unstable, and the fingers will tangle in flexion if malunion occurs.

Swelling and stiffness
These are the two enemies of rehabilitation of hand injuries: swelling leads to stiffness and stiffness prevents swelling from being pumped away, so they work together. Elevation is used to reduce swelling as quickly as possible, and movement is also started as soon as safe. A lively splint is useful in flexor tendon repairs as it uses an elastic band to flex the finger against the extensor tendon, in place of the repaired tendon. This allows the finger to be kept moving without any force being put through the freshly repaired flexor tendon.

Amputations
Traumatic amputations of fingers and even hands can be repaired, but only if the amputation occurred with a clean sharp cut, and the amputated parts can be put back quickly. Even then, it may be better to tidy up an amputation stump and concentrate on getting the individual back to work quickly rather than going through the months of rehabilitation needed for a re-implanted limb when the outcome may be uncertain. The exception to this rule is the **thumb** where every effort must be made to preserve as much length as possible because of its vital role in hand function.

Rehabilitation
Swelling of the hand as a result of trauma (especially crushing) can lead to stiffness and poor function of the hand. Early aggressive rehabilitation needs to be started to reduce swelling as quickly as possible and avoid the onset of stiffness in the joints of the hand.

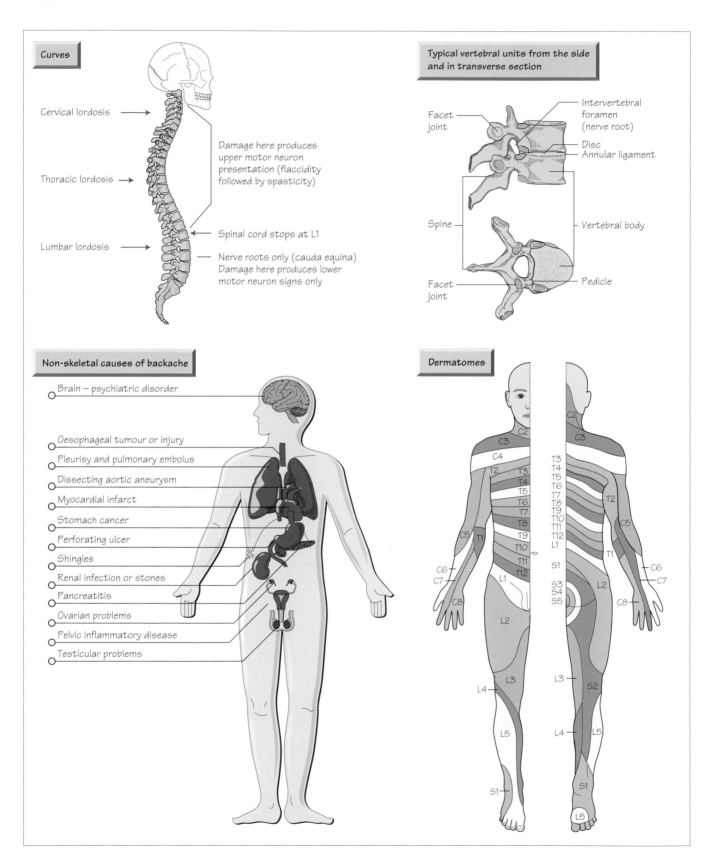

Curves

Cervical lordosis

Thoracic lordosis

Lumbar lordosis

Damage here produces upper motor neuron presentation (flaccidity followed by spasticity)

Spinal cord stops at L1

Nerve roots only (cauda equina) Damage here produces lower motor neuron signs only

Typical vertebral units from the side and in transverse section

Facet joint

Intervertebral foramen (nerve root)

Disc
Annular ligament

Spine

Vertebral body

Facet joint

Pedicle

Non-skeletal causes of backache

Brain – psychiatric disorder

Oesophageal tumour or injury

Pleurisy and pulmonary embolus

Dissecting aortic aneurysm

Myocardial infarct

Stomach cancer

Perforating ulcer

Shingles

Renal infection or stones

Pancreatitis

Ovarian problems

Pelvic inflammatory disease

Testicular problems

Dermatomes

C2
C3
C4
T2 T3
T4
T5
T6
T7
C5 T1
T8
T9
T10
C6
T11
C7
T12
L1
C8
L2

L3
L4
L5
S1

C2
C3
T3
T4
T5
T6
T7
T8
T2
T9
T10
C5
T11
T12
L1
T1
C6
C7
S1
C8
S3
S4
S5
L2

L3
S2
L4 L5
S1
L5

Function

The spine is the axial skeleton. It supports the head and the upper limbs, acts as a posterior strut for the thorax and abdomen and at its base locks into the pelvic girdle. It also acts as the conduit for nerve fibres travelling to and from the brain to the rest of the body.

Upper and lower motor neuron lesions

The upper part of the spine (above the first lumbar vertebra) also contains **spinal cord** (not just roots) and so is an extension of the **central nervous system**. Problems in this part of the spine may produce upper motor neuron signs with up-going plantar reflexes and spasticity. Below the first lumbar vertebra, obstruction of the spinal canal can only produce lower motor neuron signs, weakness and wasting combined with sensory loss.

Curves

The healthy spine has three natural curves:

1 The **cervical spine** is concave (hollow) when looked at from behind. The lowest cervical vertebra has a prominent spine which can be clearly felt and seen on X-ray.

2 The **thoracic spine** is convex.

3 The **lumbar spine** is once again hollow. The transition between the thoracic and lumbar spine is more difficult to localise.

These curves are in part a result of the shape of the bones making up the spine, but are also maintained by the tone of the muscles around the spine. Loss of, or indeed exaggeration of, these curves is suggestive of an underlying disease process.

Vertebrae

The spine is made of seven cervical, 12 thoracic and normally five lumbar vertebrae. The front part of each vertebra is solid (the body) and is the load-bearing part of the structure. Immediately behind the bodies of the vertebrae there is a hollow canal that contains the **spinal cord** (in the upper spine), but only nerve roots (the **cauda equina**) in the lumbar spine. The back wall of the canal is a thin layer of bone (the **laminae**) with a prominent crest in the midline (the **spinous process**) to which the powerful muscles running down the back of the spine are attached. At the sides, between the vertebral body and the laminae there are struts connecting the vertebral bodies to the lamellae. Arising from these **pedicles** are **facet joints** which are also joints connecting the vertebrae. Right beside these facet joints at each level there are gaps (**foraminae**) through which nerves pass out of the spinal canal. The nerves are named by the level at which they leave and are found to supply quite constant areas of skin (**dermatomes**) and muscles (**sclerotomes**).

Between the main vertebral bodies there are **intervertebral discs** – gel-filled sacks that act as shock absorbers and which, combined with the facet joints, allow a little bending and twisting between each vertebral body. When the little movement between each vertebral body is summed over the total of 24 vertebrae the flexibility of the spine in some parts is large. In the cervical spine the neck can flex and rotate. The thoracic spine is relatively rigid, while the lumbar spine falls half way between the cervical and thoracic spine.

The proximity of the spinal nerve roots to the intervertebral disc and the proximity of individual nerve roots leaving the spinal canal to the facet joint at that level makes nerve roots vulnerable to compression if either of these structures are damaged or diseased.

Trauma to the spinal cord

Significant trauma to the neck or spine usually requires quite high energy. If the displacement of the vertebrae is small, then the only injury may be tears of the ligaments or fractures and even dislocation of the facet joints. But if the displacement is greater in the upper part of the spine, then the spinal cord may be injured or even transected. Nerves in the central nervous system have a very limited power of healing and so injuries tend to be irreversible. However, things are not always as bad as they first seem, as the initial trauma to the spinal cord is accompanied by **spinal shock** (the equivalent of concussion) which wears off after some days. It is only then that the first clue to the likely severity of the permanent damage can be obtained.

Backache

Backache is common, indeed it is probably true to say that everyone has backache at some time in their lives. The problem is that it is not just the spine which can cause backache. Pancreatitis, pleurisy, a dissecting aortic aneurysm, pyelonephritis, psychiatric disorders, ovarian cysts and testicular tumours can all present with back pain, to name but a few.

To make the situation even more complicated, pathology in the back may produce pain referred to the legs or arms, or even frank neurology far from the spine in the case of nerve root entrapment. As a simple rule, always check the neck if there appears to be a problem in the upper limbs and the lumbar spine if the patient presents with problems in the legs.

11 History and examination of the spine

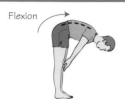

Measuring movements of the spine

Flexion

"Bend forward and try to touch your toes. Don't go further than is comfortable"

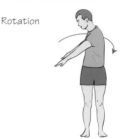

Lateral deviation

"Now slide your hand down the side of your leg, as far as it will go"

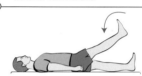

Rotation

"Keep your hips still and now twist your shoulders around as far as they will go"

Straight leg test

1. Flex up the leg – checks movement of hip joint

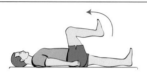

1b. Now straighten the knee letting the hip extend as little as possible

2. Check pain from tight hamstrings

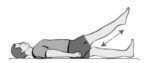

2b. Now let the hip extend 10 degrees more to relieve pain caused by tight hamstrings

3. Dorsiflexion of ankle now pulls on sciatic nerve alone

3b. Pain down the leg as the foot is dorsiflexed by the examining doctor means the test is positive

Red flags in back ache (warnings of possible severe pathology)

For fracture, infection or malignancy

History

High energy trauma
Minor injuries in people known to have osteoporosis
New episode of back pain in someone over 50 years old or under 20
Previous cancer
Generally unwell, e.g. fever, chills, unexplained weight loss
Recent infection especially urinary tract
Intravenous drug abuse
Immunosuppressed
Night pain. Pain that is worse when lying flat. Pain in the thoracic spine

Examination

Deformity

For cauda equina syndrome or rapidly progressing neurological deficit

History

Saddle anaesthesia (numbness on the inside of the thighs and around the perineum)
Recent onset of problems passing urine (e.g. urine retention, increased frequency, overflow incontinence, and inability to feel urine passing)
Recent onset of faecal incontinence

Examination

Severe or progressive loss of sensation in the lower limbs (often both)
Unexpected laxity of the anal sphincter when a rectal examination is performed
Perianal/perineal sensory loss
Major motor weakness: knee extension, ankle plantar eversion, foot dorsiflexion

Yellow flags (significant psychological component in back ache)

Belief that backache is harmful and/or potentially disabling
Fear/avoidance behaviour and reduced activity levels
Low mood and withdrawal from social interaction
Passivity in approach to treatment

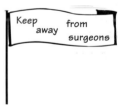

Keep away from surgeons

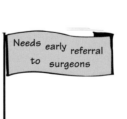

Needs early referral to surgeons

Cauda equina

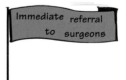

Immediate referral to surgeons

History

All patients must have had **backache** at some time in their lives. Check with them how this episode differs from any others, as this may reveal signs of sinister causes such as infection, fracture, tumour or critical nerve damage. The warning signs in the history and examination are called '**red flags**' and are designed to alert you to sinister pathology. '**Yellow flags**' are features that suggest that a psychological approach to the management of the backache will be more useful than a standard organic one (see diagram).

Examination

Exposure

The **cervical spine** can only be seen if the patient's hair is well out of the way. The bottom of the spine can be hidden by the top of the trousers. In trauma it is critical that the whole spine is examined, but the patient must be turned carefully (log-rolled) to avoid causing any further damage to the spinal cord in patients who may have an unstable fracture dislocation of the spine.

Look

Check for the normal curves of the spine and that there are no lateral curves. A hairy dimple at the base of the spine (hidden by the top of the pants) may indicate a partial failure of closure of the spinal canal (**spina bifida occulta**) which can trap nerve roots. If there is a lateral curve of the spine and it vanishes when the patient sits on the couch, then the curve is probably caused by **unequal leg lengths**. If the curve gets worse as the patient bends forward (producing a rib-hump) then it is likely to be an **idiopathic scoliosis**.

Feel

The spine can be felt through its length posteriorly. A full abdominal examination is important because back pain can be the presenting sign of many non-orthopaedic problems. Sensory loss as a result of a spine problem will be most likely in the legs or in the perineum (see section on central discs, p. 32).

Move

Examination of spinal movement is best performed with the patient standing wherever possible.
• **Flexion** of the spine can be checked by asking the patient to touch their toes. The examiner should have the tip of their thumb on the top of the lumbar spine and the index finger on the lumbosacral junction, so that the actual movement of the spine (not just flexion of the hips) can be recorded.
• **Lateral deviation** can be tested by asking the patient to slide the flats of their hands down their thighs.
• **Rotation** can be checked by holding the patient's pelvis still and then asking them to bend and look over their shoulders.

Straight leg raise test

Pain in the back commonly radiates down the leg and so can be difficult to distinguish from pain arising from the hip and knee. The straight leg raise test is designed to do this.
• The patient lies on their back and first the hip is flexed up with the knee flexed too. If there is no pain during this manoeuvre then it is unlikely that any pain is arising from the hip or knee.
• The knee is then straightened and most patients will then experience pain in the back of the thigh as the hamstring muscles tighten.
• The leg is then gently extended until the hamstrings are relaxed and the patient is again pain-free. At this point the ankle is firmly dorsiflexed. If this reproduces the back pain running down the leg it is assumed that the sciatic nerve roots are trapped as they leave the spinal canal, and the test is recorded as positive.

Reflexes and muscle power

The decision as to whether a nerve root is trapped is a critical one to the success of spine surgery. Sensory and motor loss at the same nerve level confirmed by imaging evidence of entrapment of that root as it exits the spinal canal is a very good prognosticator for the success of surgery. The knee reflex is mainly served by the L4 nerve root, while the muscle extensor hallucis longus is exclusively supplied by the L5 nerve root. The ankle reflex is mainly mediated through the S1 nerve root. These tests are therefore useful for defining the level of a lesion.

> ## Tips
>
> • Every one gets backache – most gets better spontaneously
> • Backache can arise from a multitude of different sources
> • Symptoms in the arms can arise from problems in the neck
> • Symptoms in the legs can arise from problems in the lumbar spine
> • The spinal cord only extends down to L1 so problems in the spine below this level only produce lower motor neuron signs

Problems presenting in the spine

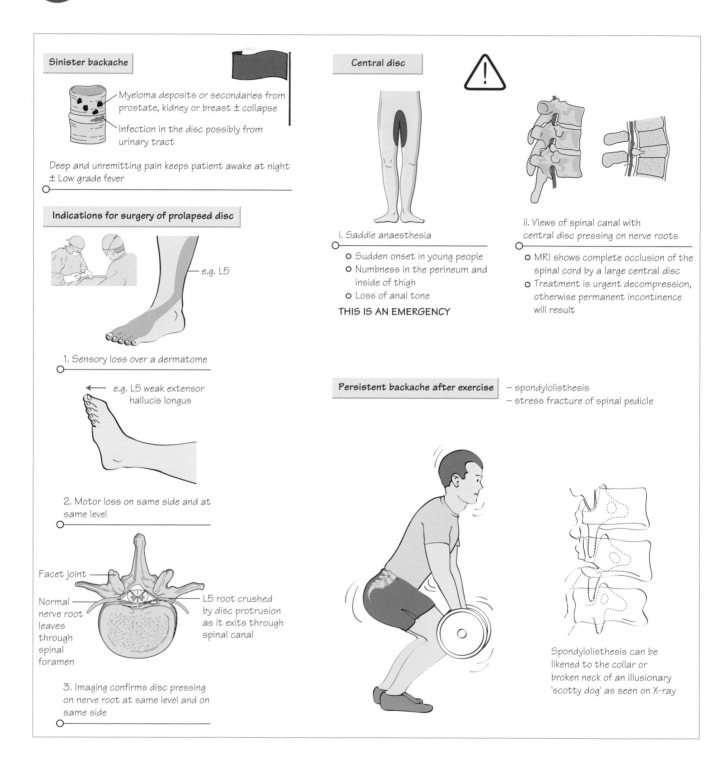

Sinister backache

Myeloma deposits or secondaries from prostate, kidney or breast ± collapse

Infection in the disc possibly from urinary tract

Deep and unremitting pain keeps patient awake at night ± Low grade fever

Indications for surgery of prolapsed disc

e.g. L5

1. Sensory loss over a dermatome

e.g. L5 weak extensor hallucis longus

2. Motor loss on same side and at same level

Facet joint

Normal nerve root leaves through spinal foramen

L5 root crushed by disc protrusion as it exits through spinal canal

3. Imaging confirms disc pressing on nerve root at same level and on same side

Central disc

i. Saddle anaesthesia

o Sudden onset in young people
o Numbness in the perineum and inside of thigh
o Loss of anal tone

THIS IS AN EMERGENCY

ii. Views of spinal canal with central disc pressing on nerve roots

o MRI shows complete occlusion of the spinal cord by a large central disc
o Treatment is urgent decompression, otherwise permanent incontinence will result

Persistent backache after exercise
– spondylolisthesis
– stress fracture of spinal pedicle

Spondylolisthesis can be likened to the collar or broken neck of an illusionary 'scotty dog' as seen on X-ray

Neck
Function
The neck is highly mobile. It is highly susceptible to injury because the weight of the head creates large forces in high energy accidents. Paradoxically, loss of mobility (stiffness) in the neck is functionally not very disabling. This is lucky because it is very common.

Presentation
• **Cervical spondylosis (arthritis)** presents with stiffness and painful spasm in the neck muscles. However, there can also be numbness and pain running down the arm. If the cause is shown to be nerve roots trapped by osteophytes, and the symptoms are disabling, surgery may need to be considered.

Whenever you see a patient with a problem in the upper limb, examine the neck as this may give you a key to the origin of the problem.

- **Rheumatoid arthritis.** In rheumatoid arthritis, the facet joints may be eroded away to such an extent that the neck becomes unstable. When a patient is anaesthetised, the neck muscles can no longer protect the neck, and the spinal cord may be damaged at intubation. It is therefore important to always inform an anaesthetist of a patient with rheumatoid arthritis so that they can ensure that suitable precautions are taken.

Thoracic spine
Function

The thoracic spine is a support for the neck and upper limbs. It moves very little apart from allowing the ribs to move and the lungs to expand during inspiration.

Presentation

- **Crush fractures** can occur in osteoporotic patients after a fall. Myeloma and secondaries can produce lytic lesions, which may also collapse.
- **Shingles.** Herpes zoster (shingles) may cause severe pain in the dermatome of an intercostal nerve.
- **Ankylosing spondylitis** may produce severe stiffness of the spine, which restricts vital capacity and may also cause a progressive flexion deformity. The latter may become so severe that the patient can no longer raise their head to look forward.
- **Scoliosis** is commonly a growth abnormality of the spine, which develops during adolescence in children of tall parents who are growing fast. It leads to rotation and then curvature of the spine, which produces a characteristic hunchback. It is much more noticeable as soon as the child bends forward to touch their toes. If the curvature looks as if it is going to become severe, surgery may be needed to straighten and fuse the spine, limiting the deformity.

Causes of backache

- **Simple mechanical low back pain.** Low back pain or **lumbago** is a vicious circle of muscle spasm creating pain, which in turn creates more muscle spasm. Most backache will get better whatever you do, but alternative medicine is useful because it seems to be good at breaking the pain cycle.
- **Sciatica.** If pain only radiates as far as the knee, then it is usually assumed that this is referred pain (the origin is in the back). If, however, the pain goes beyond the knee, down into the foot, then it is likely that this is nerve root irritation, possibly caused by a prolapsed intervertebral disc.
- **Sinister backache.** Backache that keeps patients awake at night may be due to an infection (**discitis**) or a tumour (**myeloma** or a secondary). It is usually associated with a low grade fever, and the patient feels generally unwell.
- **Prolapsed intervertebral disc.** If the contents of the disc, the nucleus pulposus, prolapse through a rupture in the annulus (the tough ring enclosing the pulposus), then there may be pressure and rubbing of the nerve roots and an inflammatory reaction may be set up. This causes **sciatica**. In over 90% of cases the inflammation dies down in time. Therefore, the condition should be allowed to take its natural course if possible. The patient will need pain relief – any measure that might help with the muscle spasm, such as osteopathy, acupuncture, aromatherapy, etc., can be used.

The **straight leg raise test** will be positive (as the nerve roots are irritated). If a patient has sensory loss or motor weakness in the distribution of a lumbar root, then they need urgent referral to an orthopaedic surgeon, where a decision can be made about whether decompression is appropriate to save the compressed nerve. The commonest nerve roots to be affected are L5 and S1.

- **Spondylolisthesis.** In this condition, a fracture occurs in the pedicles of the L5 vertebra, allowing it to slip forward on the sacrum. On examination a step is palpable at the base of the spine. It produces backache and, if the slip is severe, there may even be sciatica with nerve root compression. Treatment is difficult as the slip cannot be reduced easily. Physiotherapy may help reduce the pain. If surgery is considered the goal is limited to fusing the vertebrae so that the slip does not proceed further.

Central prolapse of the disc
History

In young people (especially women just after having children), an intervertebral disc may rupture quite suddenly and without warning. It may then extrude all its contents into the spinal canal in one catastrophic event. There may be no pain, because there is no time for the nerve roots to become inflamed, so the presentation may not be like other prolapsed intervertebral discs. Instead the patient experiences numbness down the inside of both legs (the sensory distribution of the sacral nerve roots) and may have the peculiar feeling of not knowing when they are passing urine or opening their bowels, as well as being frankly incontinent (see section on red flags, Chapter 11).

Examination

On examination the patient will have numbness around the perineum and the inside of the thigh (**saddle anaesthesia**). Anal tone may be absent on rectal examination (**patulous anus**), so the patient is not able to contract the anal sphincter onto the examiner's finger. Straight leg raise may be reduced and if it is then it is bilateral.

Investigation and treatment

This is a surgical emergency and, even if decompression is undertaken within hours, the patient may be left permanently incontinent. Luckily the condition is rare, but when it does occur, urgent action must be taken.

Immediate surgery is needed to relieve the pressure on the nerve roots. The sooner the pressure is relieved, the better the chance of a good recovery being made.

> ## Tips
>
> - Rheumatoid patients with neck involvement need care when being intubated
> - Most simple mechanical backache gets better on its own
> - Evidence of nerve root compression requires investigation
> - Backache at night may be due to an infection or tumour
> - Alternative medicine relieves the pain cycle caused by muscle spasm
> - Central disc prolapse is a true surgical emergency
> - Saddle anaesthesia and loss of anal tone are diagnostic of central disc prolapse
> - Urgent imaging and decompression offer the only hope of recovery from central disc prolapse

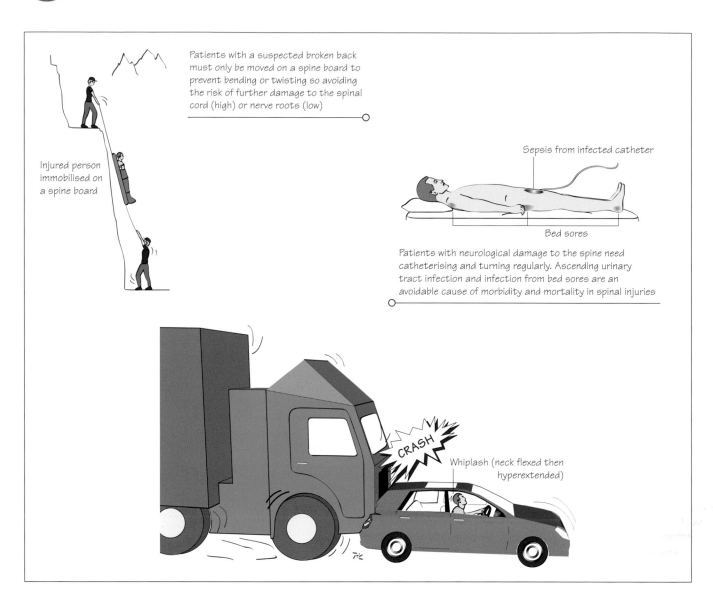

Patients with a suspected broken back must only be moved on a spine board to prevent bending or twisting so avoiding the risk of further damage to the spinal cord (high) or nerve roots (low)

Injured person immobilised on a spine board

Sepsis from infected catheter

Bed sores

Patients with neurological damage to the spine need catheterising and turning regularly. Ascending urinary tract infection and infection from bed sores are an avoidable cause of morbidity and mortality in spinal injuries

CRASH

Whiplash (neck flexed then hyperextended)

Introduction

- Problems with spine trauma can vary from a back sprained when lifting, through to permanent paralysis as a result of transection of the cord.
- Most serious spinal injuries are avoidable. Tougher safety regulations in heavy industries like mining, compulsory seat belts, roll-over bars on tractors and stricter rules in sport have all contributed to a dramatic fall in the number of these injuries in the developed world.
- All unconscious patients and any patient involved in a high energy accident should be assumed to have a spinal injury until otherwise proven. These cases are therefore best transferred to hospital on a spine board with extra protection for the cervical spine.

Minor injuries

Most people will experience **backache** at least once in their life as a result of trauma. After the initial injury the bulk of the pain is thought to come from muscle spasm, so any method that can break the vicious cycle of spasm causing pain which causes further spasm, will bring symptomatic relief. This could involve physiotherapy and/or the use of simple analgesics such as paracetamol with ibuprofen. Alternative medicine such as osteopathy, chiropractic and acupuncture can all help by reducing the pain arising from muscle spasm.

Whiplash

This is a little understood but very common condition in the neck and back of patients who have suffered spinal trauma. The classic presentation is following a car crash where the patient has been struck from behind and the neck has presumably been first hyperextended and then hyperflexed by the energy of the impact. The condition can be late in onset and may affect the head (giving **occipital headaches**), the jaw (affecting the **temporomandibular joint**), the ear (producing **tinnitus**) and even the eyes (producing **migraine-like symptoms**). It usually settles over a period of months, but has a poor prognosis if it persists for more than 2 years.

Crush fracture of the spine

This usually occurs in elderly osteoporotic patients who slip and land on their bottoms, sending a compressive force up the spine. The vertebrae (commonly in the thoracic zone) buckle. The fracture is stable but can cause severe pain while healing and even afterwards.

Fractures of the spine in younger people

These can be divided into those which are stable and those which are not, and those involving damage to the spinal cord or nerve roots and those where they are spared.

The extent of neurological damage can be very difficult to assess in the first instance because **spinal shock** (the equivalent of concussion) may give the appearance of a complete transection of the cord. However, the first sign of recovery may be some sparing of the sacral nerves, with return of sensation around the perineum. If there is no central sparing, then within a few days flaccid paralysis may be replaced by **spasticity**, an ominous sign that the spinal reflexes are dissociated from the higher centres.

If a spinal fracture is unstable it is now commonly felt that the spine should be stabilised whether there is neurological sparing or not. Rehabilitation will be quicker whatever the neurological outcome if the spine is stable. Stable spinal fractures may be explored if there is neurological compromise and it is felt that decompression of the spinal canal might help recovery.

Spinal fractures with significant neurological damage

- In the first days great care is taken with turning and moving the patient, at least until the spine is stable, to avoid further nerve damage.
- The bladder will not be functioning so the patient will need catheterisation under the most sterile possible conditions, as ascending **urinary tract infection** is a dangerous complication.
- The patient needs to be turned regularly to prevent **bed sores** from forming. Once they have occurred they are very difficult to heal and are another source of potential infection and septicaemia.
- From a psychological point of view the patient needs to be started into a rehabilitation programme as quickly as possible, preparing them to return to as independent a life as possible.
- Joints need to be kept mobile to avoid contractures.

Outcome of spinal injury involving neurological damage

Initial spinal shock may produce almost complete sensory loss and flaccid paralysis, but perineal sparing suggests good prognosis. Maximum recovery may take several years.

Level of lesion	Residual deficit if transection is complete
High cervical	If the patient survives, they will need a ventilator to breathe Spastic paralysis of the upper and lower limbs = quadriplegia
Low cervical	Breathing is spared Some use of the arms but the hands are worse affected
Thoracic	Upper limbs are spared but there is spastic paralysis of the legs May not be able to sit unaided
Lumbar	Should be able to sit Flaccid paralysis in the lower limbs

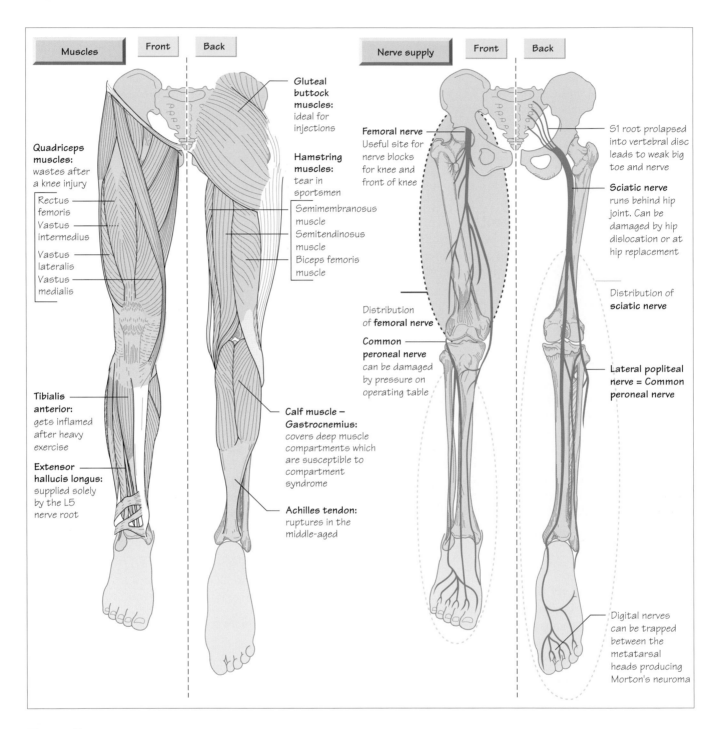

Muscles | Front | Back

Gluteal buttock muscles: ideal for injections

Hamstring muscles: tear in sportsmen

Quadriceps muscles: wastes after a knee injury

Rectus femoris
Vastus intermedius
Vastus lateralis
Vastus medialis

Semimembranosus muscle
Semitendinosus muscle
Biceps femoris muscle

Tibialis anterior: gets inflamed after heavy exercise

Extensor hallucis longus: supplied solely by the L5 nerve root

Calf muscle – Gastrocnemius: covers deep muscle compartments which are susceptible to compartment syndrome

Achilles tendon: ruptures in the middle-aged

Nerve supply | Front | Back

Femoral nerve Useful site for nerve blocks for knee and front of knee

Distribution of **femoral nerve**

Common peroneal nerve can be damaged by pressure on operating table

S1 root prolapsed into vertebral disc leads to weak big toe and nerve

Sciatic nerve runs behind hip joint. Can be damaged by hip dislocation or at hip replacement

Distribution of **sciatic nerve**

Lateral popliteal nerve = Common peroneal nerve

Digital nerves can be trapped between the metatarsal heads producing Morton's neuroma

Function

The lower limbs are designed to allow a human to move efficiently over rough ground.

• The **pelvis** acts as a platform for the spine and trunk.

• The **hip joints** are clothed in powerful muscles and have restricted movement compared with the shoulder girdle.

• The **knees** have even more restricted mobility to allow the efficient transfer of force from the foot to the body.

• The **foot** itself is light for energy-efficient movement, but nevertheless is a complex of joints, which allow the sole of the foot to grip and conform to uneven ground.

Nerves

The **femoral nerve** supplies mainly the front of the upper leg; the **sciatic nerve** supplies the back of the thigh, then the whole of the lower leg and foot. The sciatic nerve is susceptible to injury as it passes just behind the hip joint (dislocation and retractors used at joint replacement). The **peroneal nerve** can be damaged on the operating table and by obstetric stirrups.

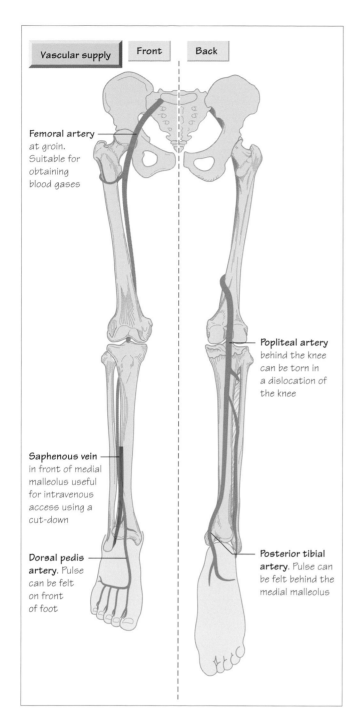

Vascular supply | Front | Back

Femoral artery at groin. Suitable for obtaining blood gases

Popliteal artery behind the knee can be torn in a dislocation of the knee

Saphenous vein in front of medial malleolus useful for intravenous access using a cut-down

Dorsal pedis artery. Pulse can be felt on front of foot

Posterior tibial artery. Pulse can be felt behind the medial malleolus

Vessels

The blood supply to the leg is mainly supplied through the **femoral artery** which passes from the groin to the back of the knee where it becomes the **popliteal artery** and then divides into three branches, two of which continue down into the foot. The popliteal artery is vulnerable to damage behind the knee due to dislocation of the knee or knee surgery.

The **long saphenous vein** is a constant feature one finger's breadth in front of and above the medial malleolus of the ankle, a useful source of venous access when all else fails.

Hip

The hip joint is a deep ball and socket, which can only develop normally if the femoral head is securely in joint. Otherwise a dysplastic or even a frankly dislocated hip develops.

The femoral head relies almost totally for its nourishment on vessels which run up through the femoral neck. If this blood supply is interrupted the femoral head has little or no capacity to recover and dies. A displaced fracture across the upper femoral neck (**sub-capital fracture**) commonly does this in the elderly, while some drugs like alcohol and steroids can also cause avascular necrosis of part or all of the femoral head in any age group.

Knee

The knee joint is especially susceptible to injury because of its rigidity and the abnormal forces applied to it in modern sport. It did not evolve to be strong enough to cope with the forces that can be generated by the use of studded boots or of skis.

The knee cap (**patella**) transmits the forces of the **quadriceps muscle** over the front of the knee. The quadriceps muscle runs in a shallow groove, which makes it susceptible to dislocation. The **cruciate ligaments** inside the knee control forward and backward glide of the femur on the tibia and are likely to be ruptured in twisting injuries. They lack an adequate blood supply to heal themselves, and can leave an athlete significantly disabled if the muscles around the knee cannot control the extra instability.

The knee, like the hip, is susceptible to developing **osteoarthritis** in the elderly, especially on the inside (medial compartment) where most of the load is taken.

Pronation and supination in the lower leg has been lost as the lower limb evolved towards being rigid for more efficient energy transmission. The **tibia** takes the vast bulk of the load; the tibia and fibula share the origins of the toe flexors and extensors.

Ankle

The ankle joint works closely with the subtalar joint to allow the foot to conform to uneven ground, and to enable the lower leg to elongate when running by allowing the foot to plantarflex. The powerful **Achilles tendon** arising from the heel and passing up to the calf muscles is the main driver of this movement.

The ankle, like the knee, is susceptible to injury because shoes enable the foot to grip the ground so securely that the forces transmitted through the bones and ligaments of the lower limb are much greater than those for which they evolved. The **fibula** makes up the lateral wall of the ankle joint and is liable to be broken if powerful twisting or bending forces pass through the ankle, such as occurs when we 'go over' on our ankle, or our body continues to turn at speed, while the foot is firmly fixed to the ground.

Foot

The foot has been in a rapid phase of evolution from a grasping organ (in tree-climbing primates) to a paw (for savannah-running hominids). However, it certainly has never had a chance to evolve to cope with shoes. The result, therefore, is that the foot is prone to many problems both in sport and as humans live longer.

Abnormal pressure and rubbing from shoes can produce **callouses** and **bone deformities** in the foot, which can be both painful and unsightly. When examining the foot do not forget to check the shoes for signs of abnormal pressure and wear. The normal-wear pattern is at the side of the heel at the back (where heel strike occurs), the outside of the shoe (transfer of load to the forefoot) and a circular wear patch under the ball of the big toe (as the forefoot pushes off).

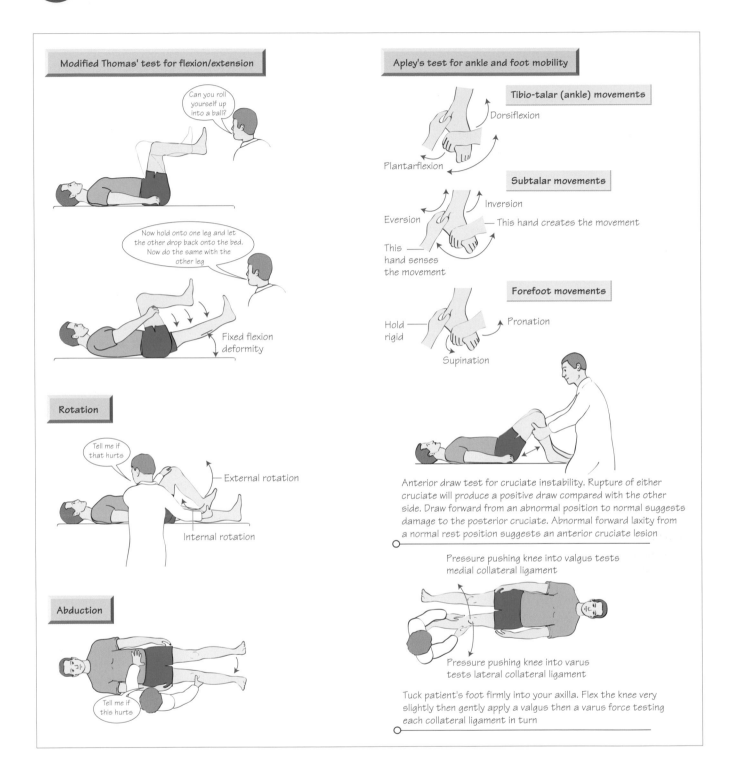

Hip

• Make sure that you have adequate exposure on both sides so that the normal can be compared with the abnormal. Use the system 'look, feel, move' (see Chapters 3, 21) and always check distal neurovascular status.

• Watch the patient walk, looking for any signs of a limp, which could be caused by pain (antalgic), weakness (Trendelenburg limp) or deformity (short). A painful hip is held flexed, adducted and internally rotated so the leg appears short.

• It is sometimes difficult to tell whether pain in the upper leg is coming from the hip, the knee or even the back. One way to exclude the hip is the 'pastry roll' test. Let the patient relax then roll the leg in and out with the flat of one hand on their thigh and the other on the shin as if you were rolling pastry. If the hip is pain-free the foot will flop too and fro at the end of the leg. If there is irritability in the hip then the patient will resist this rolling and the foot will remain rigid.

Range of movement

When checking range of movement, lie the patient on their back and then ask them to curl into a ball. Compare the flexion of the hip with the other normal side. Then, get them to use their hands to hold the normal hip in that flexed position (this fixes the position of the pelvis) and gently allow the affected hip to extend as far as is comfortable. If there is **fixed flexion deformity** the leg will not be able to extend out onto the couch (**modified Thomas' test**). When checking the range of rotation, just flex the hip enough to allow you to bend the knee to a right angle. Then use the tibia as a dial indicating the amount of rotation that can be achieved.

An **arthritic hip** usually has reduced flexion and extension (a fixed flexion deformity), a fixed adduction deformity (no abduction) and minimal rotation, especially external, of the hip joint.

Knee

The initial examination of the knee is probably best done with the patient standing so that you can inspect all sides. One of the first signs of problems in the knee is wasting of the **vastus medialis**, the muscle that bulges just above and inside the knee cap when the patient forces their knee back into hyperextension.

An **effusion** in the knee is best seen by the loss of the dimple on the inside of the knee cap when compared with the other side. The commonest bony deformity is bowing of the knees (**varus**) caused by osteoarthritis of the medial compartment.

Range of movement

Range of movement can be compared by first lifting both heels off the bed to check for loss of extension, then seeing how far up to the buttock the heel can be drawn when the patient is lying on a couch, looking for loss of flexion and comparing sides.

Stability

The **collateral ligaments** are checked by stressing the knee first into varus (inwards), then valgus (outwards), with the knee very slightly bent. It is probably easiest to sit on the couch, then tuck the patient's foot firmly into your axilla so that your hands are free to gently stress the knee first outwards into valgus (testing the medial collateral ligament) and then inwards (testing the lateral collateral). The knee needs to be very slightly flexed when performing this test as otherwise the tight posterior structures may mask collateral tenderness (a **partial tear**) or laxity (a **complete tear**).

Cruciate ligament instability is revealed by finding that the tibia is loose on the femur when pulled forward. Bend the patient's knees up to a right angle, then once again sit on the end of the couch, with the patient's feet tucked side by side under your thigh to hold them still. First look from the side to see if one tibia has sunk back on the femur (suggestive of a **ruptured posterior cruciate**). Then with both hands gripping the top of the tibia, gently try pulling it forward on the femur.

• If the distance that it will draw forward is much more than the other side, then a cruciate ligament is probably ruptured.
• If the tibia moves from a sagged back position forward to a normal position (compared with the other side) then it is the posterior cruciate ligament that is ruptured.
• If the tibia floats forward from a normal to an abnormal position, then the anterior cruciate has failed.

Pushing the patella laterally as you bend the knee will be resisted by patients who have had a previous dislocation of the knee cap (**patella apprehension sign**).

Ankle

Ankle swelling has many causes: cardiac, renal and local trauma. Local trauma will reveal tenderness that will be localised to the injured ligament or broken bones.

Range of movement

Range of movement in the ankle, the subtalar joint and the forefoot can all be checked by holding the heel in one hand and the forefoot in the other.
• Rocking the hands up and down checks plantar and dorsiflexion at the ankle joint.
• Tipping both hands in (inversion) and out (eversion) tests mobility in the subtalar joint.
• Twisting the hand holding the forefoot in (pronation) and out (supination), while holding the hindfoot still, checks movement in the small joints of the forefoot.

Foot

Check the skin all over the forefoot for bunions and corns, and on the sole of the foot for thickened pads over the metatarsal heads. Feel for tenderness in the bones and joints of the foot, checking especially whether any deformed toes can be straightened or whether the deformity is fixed.

Pathological flat feet are only reliably visible when the patient stands on their toes. A physiological flat foot (part of the normal spectrum) will form a normal arch on tip-toe. In pathological flat foot no arch forms, suggesting that there may be an abnormality in the bones of the foot. A very high arched foot is often associated with neurological problems such as spina bifida or a degenerative neurological disorder.

Tips

• Always check distal neurovascular status in lower limb problems
• Watch patients walking before starting a full examination
• Symptoms and signs in the leg can arise from problems in the spine
• The long saphenous vein can always be found one finger's breadth in front of and above the medial malleolus. A cut-down to the vein gives access if all else fails

16 Problems presenting in the hip

Septic arthritis

Premature baby (more rarely at any age)
o Toxic
o Doesn't move the affected limb
o Joint is destroyed if not treated early

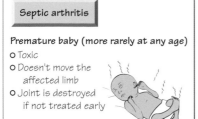

Developmental dysplasia of hip (DDH)

Newborn baby
o Congenital dislocation of the hip. If the hip is not held in joint it will develop badly (dysplastic)

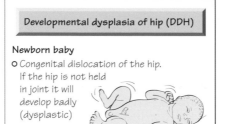

Perthe's disease

Limping child (4–10 years)
o Spontaneous avascular necrosis of the femoral head.
Needs protecting while it regrows or it will collapse

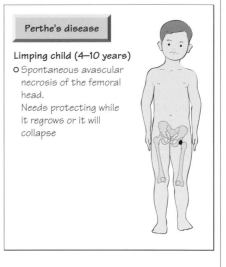

Adult hip

Normal   Dysplastic

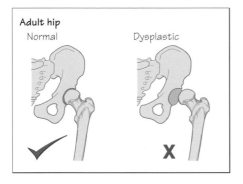

✓   X

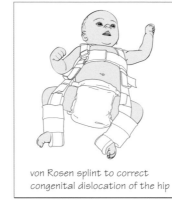

von Rosen splint to correct congenital dislocation of the hip

Slipped upper femoral epiphysis

Limping child around puberty

o Foot turns out. Leg shortens. Only clearly visible on lateral X-ray

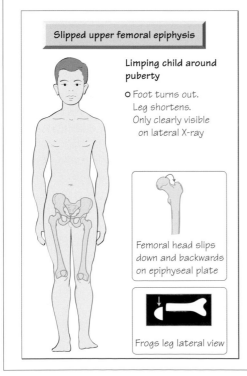

Femoral head slips down and backwards on epiphyseal plate

Frogs leg lateral view

Osteoarthritis in the elderly

Painful limp in elderly

o Cysts
o Loss of joint space
o Sclerosis around joint
o Osteophytes

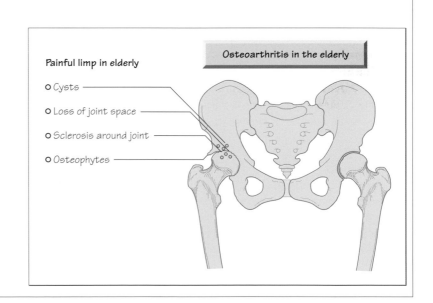

Introduction

Problems with the hip can occur at any age, and for each age group the most likely diagnosis is different.

Hip dysplasia

The condition is not common, but is most easily treated if it is spotted early. There are many associations such as family history or the child being a first born female, particularly if the delivery is breech. If there is any suspicion from the history or on examination at birth, then the diagnosis should be confirmed or excluded using a dynamic ultrasound examination of both hips. If the hip is abnormal then if it can be held in the **acetabulum**, using splints that hold the legs in abduction and external rotation, the femoral head will then grow within the acetabulum, and the hip joint will develop normally. If this treatment fails (or was never instituted), then the lack of congruence in the hip joint will result in abnormal development, which will require surgical correction later in life.

Late diagnosis of congenital dislocation of the hip

This is more common in first born girls, and in breech deliveries. When children start walking it may be noted that they are limping and that the buttock creases are asymmetrical. The most likely diagnosis is a congenital dislocation of the hip that was not spotted at birth. After the age of 6 weeks the femoral head has started to ossify, so it is possible to see that the hip is dislocated on X-ray. An ultrasound scan will also confirm the diagnosis. The key to treatment is to get the hip into the joint as soon as possible and to hold it there, so that the acetabulum and femoral head can develop congruently. Splints that hold the hip abducted may be adequate; if not surgery will be needed to clear out any soft tissue blocking reduction.

Septic arthritis

In a child too young to speak it may be difficult to work out where they are getting pain, but if the child is watched for a time it will be noticed that, however fretful they are, they do not move the painful limb. The diagnosis that must be considered is septic arthritis of the joint (see Chapter 25).

Irritable hip

Young children are frequently referred as emergencies with a limp. It can be very difficult to make the diagnosis, as they may not be able to explain why they will no longer weight bear normally on that leg. Even when they are old enough to talk and explain the problem, they frequently complain of pain in the knee when the problem is in fact in the hip.

Any child who is limping should have a careful examination of the whole leg. If the problem is in the hip then there will be painful limitation to movement of internal rotation of the hip (see p. 36). In more severe cases the hip is held flexed, internally rotated and adducted (the position of maximum comfort). Most cases of irritable hip are of unknown cause but may be some form of transient **post-viral arthritis**. The condition settles spontaneously within a few days or weeks.

Perthe's disease

In children aged 4–10 years, Perthe's disease produces a sustained irritable hip. The underlying pathology is thought to be avascular necrosis of the femoral head for no known reason (idiopathic). The femoral head will revascularise in time but if the segment of dead bone is large or the hip is subjected to a high load before it has had time to repair, then the femoral head collapses and the early onset of arthritis is inevitable. The hip should therefore be protected as much as possible during this period. Operations to protect the vulnerable segment of cartilage are of unproven value.

Slipped upper femoral epiphysis

In children around the age of puberty, the **ephiphyseal plate** seems to be especially weak. Failure of the plate leads to slip of the femoral head downwards and backwards in relation to the femoral neck. The deformity is easy to miss on an anteroposterior X-ray, but is obvious on a lateral or 'frog's leg' view. The child presents with a limp and often pain in the knee (referred pain), so the diagnosis is easy to miss. The foot is often turned outwards compared with the other side. If pins are run across the epiphysis, any further slip can be prevented until the epiphysis has fused at the end of growth. The condition is often bilateral.

Osteoarthritis of the hip

This may develop in young people as a result of trauma, inflammatory joint disease or hip dysplasia (an abnormal-shaped hip from birth). However, it is normally a disease of the elderly, causing a limp because of pain, stiffness, weakness or a shortened leg. Hip replacement is the treatment of choice (see Chapter 17), although in younger patients with dysplasia an osteotomy may be used to improve the shape of the hip and so prolong its life.

Avascular necrosis

High alcohol intake, steroids and some storage disorders predispose patients to develop avascular necrosis of the hip. The femoral head may take some years to collapse after the initial insult, but once it has collapsed a total hip replacement is the only option for restoring function and relieving pain.

> **Tips**
>
> • Exclude Perthe's disease and slipped upper femoral epiphysis in a child with a limp
> • A dislocated hip at birth will not develop properly if it is not relocated

Joint replacement

Joint replacements mainly reduce pain and can improve mobility. The chance of the operation being successful and the longevity of the implant varies between joints

Shoulder

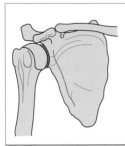

- Useful in end-stage inflammatory arthritis where they reduce pain but may not improve mobility much
- Hemi-arthroplasties replace a badly fractured humeral head
- Results variable

Wrist

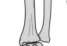

- Fusion gives a strong pain-free wrist. This is a better option than artificial wrist joints

Metacarpophalangeal joints

- Can be replaced in hands damaged by rheumatoid arthritis
- Improves cosmesis and function

Knee

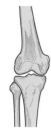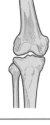

- Now as good as hip replacement in terms of reliability (Over 90% successful for more than 10 years)
- Half-knee (unicompartmental) replacements also available

Ankle

- Useful for reducing pain and improving function especially in rheumatoid arthritis
- Reliability not as good as hips and knees

Spine

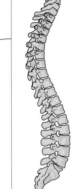

- Synthetic intervertebral discs are now available
- Short and long term value is not yet clear

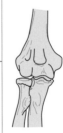

Elbow

- Good pain relief and mobility improvement in rheumatoid arthritis
- Results good
- Artificial radial head can stabilise the elbow if severity of fracture requires removal of patient's radial head

Hip

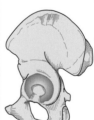

- Reliably reduce pain and improve mobility in arthritis
- Last for 10–15 years and can then be replaced (revised)
- New materials (ceramics) and new designs (surface replacement) may provide even better results but are not yet proven
- Probably over 100,000 performed every year in UK alone

Introduction

Damaged joints become stiff, weak and painful. This interferes with activities of daily living and with sleep, and can convert a person who was an outgoing and independent contributor to society into a depressive reliant on society for their needs.

Pathophysiology

Joints most commonly fail because of **idiopathic osteoarthritis** – the collapse of the articular cartilage for no known cause. However, joints can also fail as a result of the destruction caused by **destructive arthritis** or even **fractures** into the joint. If the surface of a joint heals with more than a 2 mm step in the surface, the onset of **early traumatic arthritis** is thought to be almost inevitable. Arthritic pain at night is a deep ache within the bones of the joint, while during the day the joint is stiff and hurts when it is moved.

Treatment

The options to manage the symptoms are painkillers, physiotherapy and aids to ease activities of everyday living, such as splints and home aids. Injections of local anaesthetic and even steroids into the joint give only minimal short-term benefit and run the risk of introducing infection into the joint.

Surgically the options are either to fuse the joint, excise it, or replace it:

• **Fusion** removes all movement but should create a strong limb which is pain-free.
• **Excision** should also remove pain but preserves movement although strength is lost because the muscles no longer have a fulcrum across which they can operate.
• **Replacement** should remove pain, improve mobility at least a little, and provide a strong limb.

Surprisingly, loss of mobility in the wrist is no great disability, so fusion may be the operation of choice here. Loss of strength and stability in the lateral compartment of the adult elbow is not a problem so excision of the proximal radial head is the treatment of choice in radiohumeral arthritis. In the hip or knee, joint replacement is now the treatment of choice (at least in the elderly). As techniques improve joint replacement is becoming the treatment of choice in shoulders, elbows and ankles.

Problems with artificial joints

The problem with artificial joints is first that they do not last long (not nearly as long as manufacturers would have us believe). They are also not as strong as the joint surfaces they replace and are therefore prone to breaking if the patient falls. The materials used for joint replacement are changing as we seek implants that are stronger, have lower friction and produce fewer wear particles. Implants with low friction put less load on their fixation to the bone beneath. Wear particles stimulate an inflammatory response in the joint which leads to bone resorption around the implant and therefore loosening.

Prognosis

Hip and knee replacements probably give significant pain relief for 10–15 years. Once they start to loosen, pain and instability return. At this stage it is normally possible to replace the worn-out joint with a revision implant fitted into the cleaned-out bed of the old implant. This implant does not usually last as long as a primary replacement but may give 7–10 years of useful life. Once the joint can no longer be replaced, it may need removing to reduce pain, leaving a flail but painless joint.

Complications of major joint replacements

• The death rate after joint replacement is less than one per 1000. Most of these deaths are a result of heart attacks and strokes.
• Infection and wound break down occurs in less than 2% of cases. Infection rates are held down by using prophylactic antibiotics and by using laminar flow theatres where only sterile air is allowed to flow over the patient's wound.
• A hip replacement is prone to dislocation especially in the 6 weeks after surgery before a new capsule has grown around the hip joint. This risk of around 2% can be kept to a minimum by making sure that the patient does not sit on low chairs or cross their legs during this critical period.
• A knee replacement is very painful for many weeks and is susceptible to stiffness as a result. If this cannot be overcome by exercises and physiotherapy then a manipulation under anaesthetic may be needed to break down the adhesions.
• Both hip and knee replacements can cause damage to nerves that travel close to the joint being replaced.
• In hip replacements leg length may be difficult to match with the opposite leg, and a heel raise may be needed in the patient's shoe to balance the legs up.

An **infected joint replacement** tends to present insidiously, not at all like septic arthritis. The patient has continuing pain after the joint replacement and may have a low grade fever. The wound may also be red and tender. Sometimes the first clue is bone resorption visible on X-ray. The only way to be sure of the diagnosis is to open the joint and take multiple samples. If the joint proves to be infected, and the infection is caught early, it must be washed out and the patient given high doses of intravenous antibiotics for at least 6 weeks. However, if the diagnosis is delayed, as is so often the case, the implant will need removing. A new implant cannot always be put back in, so the patient may be left without a joint.

Expectations

• Patients with successful joint replacements can return to a full, pain-free life – driving their cars, playing golf and swimming.
• Osteoarthritis appears to be a systemic disease and the replacement of one joint often exposes arthritic pain in other joints, so patients who have had one successful joint replacement often return for several more.

Shoulder, elbow, metacarpal and ankle replacements

Replacements for all these joints have now been designed and are starting to produce consistently good results. They are especially useful in patients with **rheumatoid arthritis** for whom every painless functioning joint is a huge bonus.

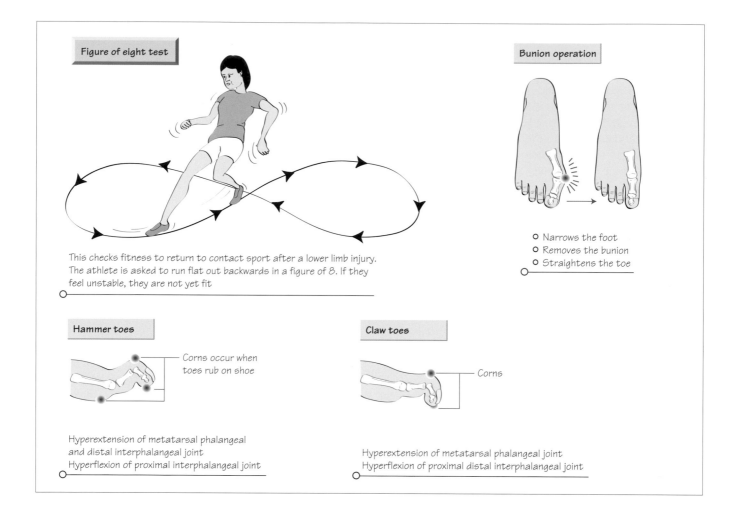

Figure of eight test

This checks fitness to return to contact sport after a lower limb injury. The athlete is asked to run flat out backwards in a figure of 8. If they feel unstable, they are not yet fit

Bunion operation

○ Narrows the foot
○ Removes the bunion
○ Straightens the toe

Hammer toes

Corns occur when toes rub on shoe

Hyperextension of metatarsal phalangeal and distal interphalangeal joint
Hyperflexion of proximal interphalangeal joint

Claw toes

Corns

Hyperextension of metatarsal phalangeal joint
Hyperflexion of proximal distal interphalangeal joint

Knee

The knee is very susceptible to problems, especially from sports such as football and skiing. The history will give a clue to the structures likely to be damaged. The key to rehabilitation of problems with the knee is physiotherapy, as the quadriceps muscle wastes very quickly if the knee has been injured. Control of knee movements is lost, and the knee is then susceptible to a secondary injury such as a tear of the meniscus. Patients with injured knees should not return to sport until the muscle has recovered. A simple test for this is to ask the athlete to run as fast as they can – backwards – in a figure of eight (**'figure of eight' test**). If the knee feels unstable to the athlete, more work is needed before they are safe to return to sport.

Locking and pseudo-locking

• **Locking** is the sensation that a patient gets when walking along and quite suddenly the knee will not straighten. The patient may end up sitting in the road jiggling the knee until the mechanical block clears from the knee. This is characteristic of a torn meniscus or of a loose body jamming in the knee.
• **Pseudo-locking** occurs in a knee which is inflamed, when the

knee is first moved after a period of stillness. This first movement causes such severe pain that the patient cannot move it further, until the inflamed layers of synovium that have stuck together are freed up. Pseudo-locking occurs commonly in teenage children, especially girls, and is associated with pain in the front of the knee and great difficulty on stairs especially descending. This anterior inflammation of the knee is sometimes called **chondromalacia patellae** (a beautiful but meaningless name) and usually resolves spontaneously.

Patella apprehension

Hypermobile patients are liable to dislocate the knee cap laterally. Once this occurs, any attempt to reproduce the dislocation (by pushing the knee cap laterally, as the knee is flexed) produces an 'impending sense of doom' in the patient similar to the shoulder apprehension sign (see Chapter 6).

Anterior cruciate tear

The anterior cruciate ligament stops the tibia sliding forward and rotating on the femur. It is torn by a twisting injury on a bent knee. It has no blood supply and so cannot heal. If the quadriceps cannot be built up enough to control the knee, then the patient will find the knee giving way when they twist or turn on it. The abnormal movement in the knee often leads to a tear of the menisci as well, causing true locking. The torn menisci need repairing or trimming through the arthroscope, and if the patient cannot cope with the instability even after intensive physiotherapy, then a substitute anterior cruciate ligament may need to be inserted, followed by a long course of rebuilding strength and proprioception around the knee.

Arthritis in the knee

This is as common in the elderly as arthritis of the hip. The patient gets pain at the end of the day and at night. There may be a lump at the back of the knee (**Baker's cyst**) – an outpouching of the excess synovial fluid. Total knee replacements can now give as reliable results as hip replacements, lasting 10–15 years before wearing out and needing changing. Osteoarthritis normally starts in the medial tibiofemoral joint so there are sometimes indications for a unicompartmental knee replacement (just one-half of the joint).

Ankle
Instability

Chronic instability of the ankle can arise after a torn ligament fails to heal. Surgical repair with a substitute ligament, followed by intensive physiotherapy, should offer reasonable results.

Arthritis of the ankle

This is common after trauma involving the ankle and in patients with inflammatory joint disease. Ankles are best fused if there is osteoarthritis or arthritis secondary to trauma, as ankle replacements tend not to do well in these conditions. However ankle replacements do well in patients with inflammatory joint disease and are especially useful because other joints around the ankle affected by the same disease are likely to be stiff.

Foot
Bunions

These are very common especially in people with wide feet who try to wear narrow shoes. The big toe bends laterally leaving a prominent head of the metatarsal bone which forms a bursa over it while the skin becomes inflamed. Surgery is designed to narrow the foot with an osteotomy through the metatarsal, while at the same time the bunion itself is removed and the toe straightened.

Claw toes, hammer toes and metatarsalgia

• Inflammatory joint disease in the feet causes dorsal dislocation of the metatarsal phalangeal joints with clawing of the toes. The metatarsal heads become very tender to walk on. Patients often describe a feeling as of walking barefoot over pebbles (**metatarsalgia**). Operations to straighten the toes and bring a thick pad of tissue over the metatarsal heads, combined with properly padded shoes, can make walking much more comfortable.
• Hammer toes result from spasm, then contracture of the intrinsic muscles of the foot.
• Patients with rheumatoid arthritis are especially susceptible to problems in the feet because of the disease's affinity for the small joints in the hand and foot.

Flat feet

Some people have a high arch to the foot, others a lower one, but true flat foot is a failure of the foot to form an arch when the patient stands on their toes (the **windlass test**). It can be caused by **congenital tarsal coalition** (bones fused from birth) or occurs in patients with inflammatory arthritis where the ligaments supporting the arch have stretched out. Pathological flat feet are difficult to treat either non-operatively with special shoes or surgically with tendon transfers or joint fusion operations.

Tips

• The figure of eight test is useful for telling when an athlete is ready to return to sport
• Locking of the knee suggests a torn cartilage; pseudo-locking may be inflammation only
• Osteoarthritis of the ankle is best treated with fusion; rheumatoid arthritis with a replacement
• Arthritis and deformity in the foot is common and disabling

19 Upper leg trauma

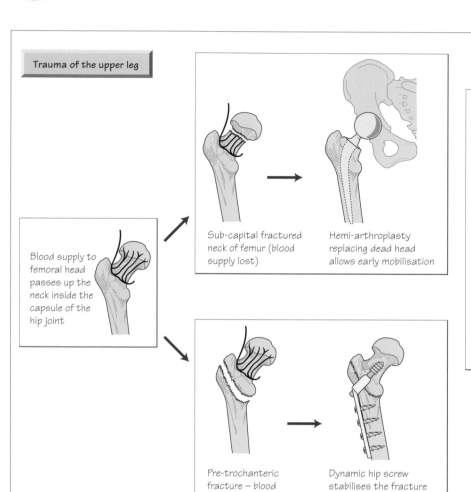

Trauma of the upper leg

Blood supply to femoral head passes up the neck inside the capsule of the hip joint

Sub-capital fractured neck of femur (blood supply lost)

Hemi-arthroplasty replacing dead head allows early mobilisation

Pre-trochanteric fracture – blood supply preserved

Dynamic hip screw stabilises the fracture allowing early mobilisation

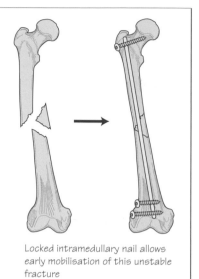

Locked intramedullary nail allows early mobilisation of this unstable fracture

Fracture of the pelvis

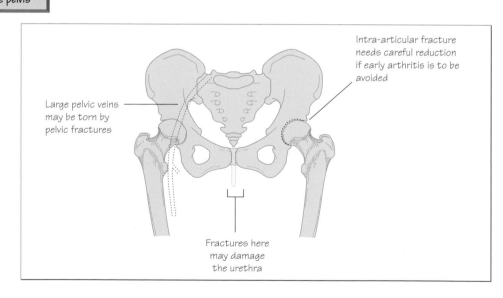

Large pelvic veins may be torn by pelvic fractures

Intra-articular fracture needs careful reduction if early arthritis is to be avoided

Fractures here may damage the urethra

Fractures of the femur

One of the most common but potentially disastrous fractures of the elderly is a fractured neck of the femur, a result of **osteoporosis**. Treatment includes the patient's rehabilitation into the community, not just the surgery itself. Otherwise the fall and the fracture (whichever came first) may be the 'straw that breaks the camel's back', condemning an elderly person living independently to a life in care or even premature death.

Sub-capital and per-trochanteric fractured neck of the femur

The blood supply to the head of the femur runs up the neck of the femur from a rim where the capsule of the hip joint attaches to the base of the neck of the femur. If the fracture is a sub-capital fractured neck of the femur, high under the head, then, in the elderly, the blood supply to the head is usually so badly compromised that even if the fracture is reduced, the head will die. The only choice in this case is to replace the femoral head. The acetabulum is not affected so only one-half of the joint is replaced. This is called a **hemi-arthroplasty**.

However, if the fracture is outside the insertion of the capsule at the base of the neck or even through the greater and lesser trochanter, the blood supply to the femoral head is unaffected. However, the fracture is very unstable, so it is usually fixed with a large screw inserted up the femoral neck, which is then attached to a plate fixed to the outside of the upper femur using screws. This system of fixation is called a **dynamic hip screw** because the screw impaling the neck and head of the femur can slip down onto the plate fixed to the upper femur allowing the fracture to compress and bed down. This improves the strength of the fixation and encourages early healing.

Both methods of fixation for the two types of fracture relieve pain and allow the patient to mobilise at once. This minimises the risk of all the complications of confining an elderly person to bed, such as bedsores, and chest and urinary tract infection. Most importantly it also helps them psychologically by enabling them to get home before they have lost their will for independent existence.

High velocity fractures

Fractures of the pelvis and of the shaft of the femur in young people are usually high velocity injuries, so other injuries need to be excluded.
• **Pelvic fractures** are notorious for catastrophic haemorrhage and for damage to the urinogenital tract. Fixation of unstable fractures of the pelvis is very difficult.
• **Femoral shaft fractures** are best fixed with a plate or an intramedullary nail so that the patient can be discharged and return to normal life as quickly as possible. The same applies to fractures of the femur through metastases in the elderly, but in this case radiotherapy will also be used to prevent local recurrence.

Knee

Injuries to the knee usually involve damage to the soft tissue, tearing of a meniscus or the rupture of a cruciate ligament. The patella can commonly dislocate laterally, but the knee itself rarely dislocates except in severe trauma. If this occurs, the popliteal artery can be damaged. A check of distal neurovascular deficit will identify what is now the real surgical emergency. The patella can be fractured by excessive force on the extensor mechanism (transverse), or by a direct blow which produces a stellate (multifragment fracture). Fractures of the femoral condyles or of the tibial plateau usually involve high energy trauma. If early post-traumatic arthritis is to be avoided the joint surface must be reconstructed so that there are no steps of more than 2 mm in the surface. This usually requires complex internal fixation with plates and screws and bone graft to fill the defect in the bone.

Torn meniscus (cartilage)

There are two menisci in each knee helping transmit load from the curved medial and lateral femoral condyles to the flat top of the tibia. The menisci have no blood or nerve supply. If they are trapped in an abnormal position they can split, and jam in the joint. The unstable fragment of the meniscus may cause no symptoms for long periods, but from time to time it may jam in the joint, producing locking. This produces a sudden onset of pain in the joint, which locks in one position. The patient may find that after a period of wiggling the knee, the unstable fragment returns to its normal position and the knee then functions normally again. The diagnosis can be made with MRI or at arthroscopy, when the offending fragment can be trimmed back.

Torn cruciate ligament

If the body of an athlete turns rapidly on a fixed foot, the loads on the knee are enormous. It is the anterior cruciate ligament which is commonly ruptured. The knee is now potentially unstable especially when turning on a bent knee and is liable to give way. Intensive physiotherapy to build up the muscles controlling the knee can often provide enough control for an athlete to manage without their cruciate ligament. If not, then a substitute anterior cruciate ligament can be inserted, but it is difficult to find any material strong enough to withstand the forces that go through this ligament, so surgery is not always successful.

Rehabilitation

The key to recovery of knee function is physiotherapy designed to:
• Build up the strength of the muscles around the knee, especially the quadriceps.
• Retrain the athlete in control (proprioception) of the knee, so that the muscles can protect the ligaments from excessive load.

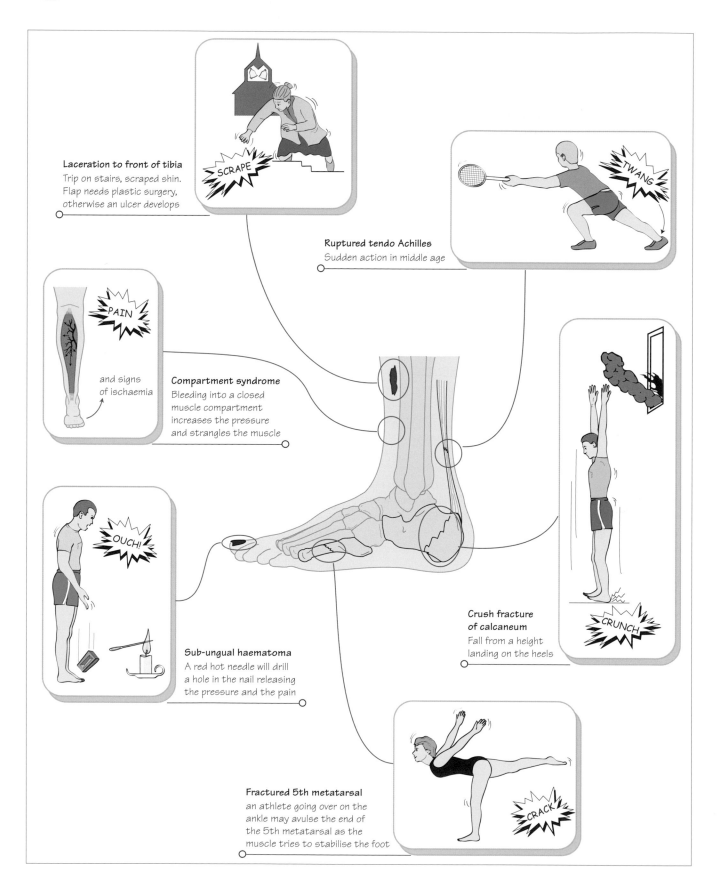

Laceration to front of tibia
Trip on stairs, scraped shin. Flap needs plastic surgery, otherwise an ulcer develops

SCRAPE

TWANG

Ruptured tendo Achilles
Sudden action in middle age

PAIN

and signs of ischaemia

Compartment syndrome
Bleeding into a closed muscle compartment increases the pressure and strangles the muscle

OUCH!

Crush fracture of calcaneum
Fall from a height landing on the heels

CRUNCH

Sub-ungual haematoma
A red hot needle will drill a hole in the nail releasing the pressure and the pain

Fractured 5th metatarsal
an athlete going over on the ankle may avulse the end of the 5th metatarsal as the muscle tries to stabilise the foot

CRACK

Introduction

Trauma of the lower leg is common, both as a result of sports and because of accidents at work. 'Going over' on the ankle can simply result in a mild ligamentous sprain, but as the energy involved in the injury rises there is a well defined cascade of fractures and ligament tears associated with each mechanism of injury. **Dislocation of the ankle** is an emergency because the pressure from the displaced talus compromises the blood supply to the foot and the integrity of the skin that is tented over the bone. Immediate reduction, even if a proper anaesthetic is not available, is appropriate because the neurovascular state of the foot is compromised.

High energy injuries

These are commonly associated with contact sports, motor vehicle crashes or falls.

• **Fractures of the tibia** are now best treated with internal fixation in most cases, as they are slow to heal without support and may require long periods in plaster. Fractures of the tibia are associated with compartment syndrome in the deep compartments (see Chapter 41).

• **Ankle fractures** need careful reconstruction to ensure that the joint surfaces are congruent, otherwise early arthritis is inevitable. The distal tibia and fibula are held together by a ligament crossing this diastasis. If this ligament is torn the stability of the ankle joint is lost and unless it is repaired, the instability will lead to early arthritis. Even if the ankle joint is internally fixed the repair will need protecting with a below-knee plaster extending to the toes. It is important that this plaster is applied with the ankle dorsiflexed at least to neutral. If the foot is plastered with the toes pointing down, the ankle stiffens in this position and is very difficult to correct later.

• **Falls from a height** can cause a string of fractures through the body, from crush fractures of the vertebrae, through fractures of the pelvis, crush fractures of the tibial plateau at the knee and the plafond at the ankle, and finally fractures of the calcaneum which can extend into the subtalar joint.

Lower energy injuries

• On examination of a simple **sprain of the ankle** there will be swelling and tenderness over the injured ligament but no tenderness over the bone itself. A below-knee plaster is only needed for comfort in the short term, otherwise the injury should be managed using RICE (see Chapter 31). Physiotherapy is also important to retrain proprioception around the ankle joint otherwise repeated injuries are likely to occur.

• **Inversion of the ankle** is controlled by the tendons passing down into the lateral side of the foot. The force generated by these tendons can pull off a fragment of bone where they insert. The classic one of these is avulsion of the proximal end of the fifth metatarsal bone. Surprisingly, it heals well without aggressive intervention.

• The **Achilles tendon** is important for transferring energy through the ankle into the ground. In the middle-aged (as collagen starts to degrade) it is liable to sudden rupture during strenuous sport. The patient may still be able to stand on their toes (using other muscles) but physical examination and, if necessary, ultrasound will confirm the diagnosis. Healing is very slow because of the poor blood supply, but surgery is also difficult because it is difficult to make a strong repair. Either way, rehabilitation is a slow and delicate balance between going too slow and risking stiffness, and going too fast and causing re-rupture.

Degloving injuries

The foot or leg can be degloved by a run-over injury. Work boots with steel toecaps are now mandatory in any high-risk work area to prevent these injuries. Initially the injury may look minor and X-rays may show no broken bones. However, the skin will have no sensation and capillary filling will be compromised. When all the dead soft tissues are removed (as they must be), the extent of the injury may make immediate **amputation** the most obvious choice.

A less severe but more common injury is a flap lifted from the front of the shin where an elderly person has tripped and barked their shin on the edge of a step. The temptation to stitch the flap back should be resisted. It is usually not viable and the swelling against tight stitches will seal its fate. Immediate plastic surgical treatment with grafting may prevent the formation of a large leg ulcer which may take many months to heal.

Fractured toes

These rarely need reducing unless they are also dislocated. Buddy strapping (bandaging to the next uninjured toe) is valuable in treating both fractured toes and simple fractures of the fingers as it provides support while allowing mobility.

Subungual haematoma

A bruise forming under a nail can be disproportionately painful. Decompression by making a hole in the nail with a red hot needle is a surprisingly painless procedure, and provides dramatic and immediate pain relief.

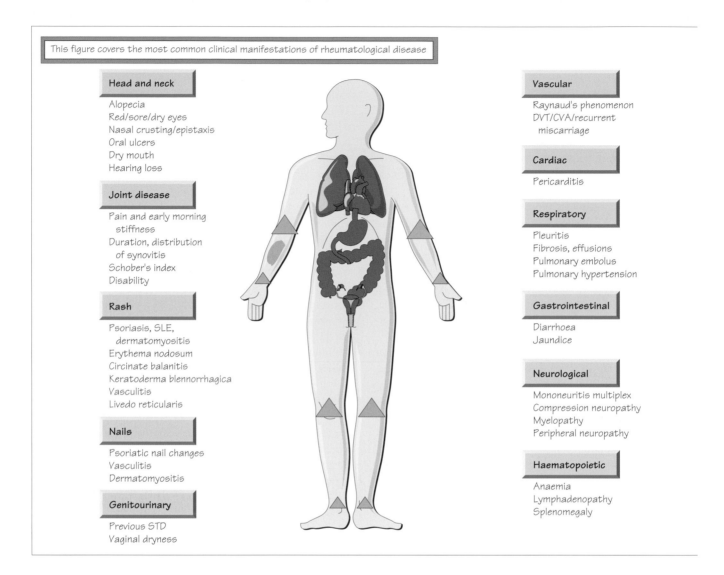

This figure covers the most common clinical manifestations of rheumatological disease

Head and neck

Alopecia
Red/sore/dry eyes
Nasal crusting/epistaxis
Oral ulcers
Dry mouth
Hearing loss

Joint disease

Pain and early morning
   stiffness
Duration, distribution
   of synovitis
Schober's index
Disability

Rash

Psoriasis, SLE,
   dermatomyositis
Erythema nodosum
Circinate balanitis
Keratoderma blennorrhagica
Vasculitis
Livedo reticularis

Nails

Psoriatic nail changes
Vasculitis
Dermatomyositis

Genitourinary

Previous STD
Vaginal dryness

Vascular

Raynaud's phenomenon
DVT/CVA/recurrent
   miscarriage

Cardiac

Pericarditis

Respiratory

Pleuritis
Fibrosis, effusions
Pulmonary embolus
Pulmonary hypertension

Gastrointestinal

Diarrhoea
Jaundice

Neurological

Mononeuritis multiplex
Compression neuropathy
Myelopathy
Peripheral neuropathy

Haematopoietic

Anaemia
Lymphadenopathy
Splenomegaly

History

The musculoskeletal history has the same basic framework as any medical or surgical history with details of the presenting complaint, history of presenting complaint, etc. There are, however, a number of features that should be highlighted when clerking and presenting a patient with rheumatological disease.

• The most crucial element in a musculoskeletal history is to differentiate inflammatory and degenerative joint disease:

   Inflammatory joint disease such as rheumatoid arthritis (RA) is characterised by the presence of *stiffness* after periods of immobility that improves with activity; *early morning* exacerbation of symptoms is classic.

   Degenerative joint disease may produce a 'gelling' sensation on waking but the problem is short lived and in general the pain is activity-related and improves with rest.

• **Joint swelling** may occur with either inflammatory or degenerative disease. The detection of swelling, its character and distribution forms the basis of clinical examination.

• **Extra-articular disease** is a frequent phenomenon in inflammatory conditions. Seeking examples of eye, skin and nail, respiratory or bowel symptoms may help not only in determining the underlying diagnosis but also its severity.

• Heritability plays a variable role in inflammatory disease and a *family history* of joint disease, psoriasis or autoimmune disease may be relevant.

• A *summary of medications* past and present is crucial. The efficacy, tolerability and patient's compliance with anti-inflammatories, disease-modifying antirheumatic drugs (DMARDs) or immunosuppressives is extremely helpful. A full alcohol and drug history is particularly pertinent in the assessment of a patient with gout.

• The degree of disability does not always correlate with the severity of joint deformity, so a full *social history* with particular attention to reports of work absenteeism and/or ability to self-care is mandatory.

Examination

The purpose of joint examination is the detection of joint swelling, differentiation between inflammatory and degenerative joint disease and the assessment of disease activity in an individual patient.

• Joint swelling in inflammation (**synovitis**) is *boggy* in nature. The joint is often *warm*, with overlying **erythema** and there is often pain at the extremes of movement. Swelling due to degenerative disease is bony hard.

• Different inflammatory diseases have predilections for different sites. Rheumatoid arthritis, for example, favours the metacarpophalangeal (MCP) and proximal interphalangeal (PIP) joints in the hand, with relative sparing of the distal interphalangeal (DIP) joints. However, osteoarthritis in the hand focuses on the first carpometacarpal (CMC) joint, the PIP joints (forming **Bouchard's nodes**) and the DIP joints (forming **Heberden's nodes**). The classic distribution for each inflammatory joint disease is covered in individual chapters.

• Many rheumatological conditions are systemic diseases. Potential extra-articular manifestations of disease must be sought in clinical examination.

The GALS screen and detailed examination of the arm, leg and spine has already been described (see Chapter 3). The rest of this chapter is therefore devoted to examination of the hand, which follows the same paradigm of 'look, feel, move'. For RA patients, the focus is not only the description of the classic bony deformity but also the detection of active synovitis (swollen and tender joints).

Look

• Stand back and take an overall view of the patient:
  Well or not?
  Stigmata of steroid use?
• Ask the patient to roll up their sleeves and show you their elbows:
  Glimpse of hand function/disability
  Check extensor surface for rheumatoid nodules or psoriatic plaques.

• Place the patient's hands palm down on a pillow:
  Skin – Stigmata of steroid use? Erythema? Rash? Scars? Vasculitic lesions?
  Nails – Psoriatic nail changes? Nail bed changes of connective disease?
  Soft tissue – Swelling? Rheumatoid nodules? Muscle wasting?
  Bone – Swelling? Classic rheumatoid changes?
• Ask the patient to lift their hands, straighten their fingers and turn their hands over:
  Extensor tendons intact? Evidence of wrist restriction?
• Place patient's hands palm up on a pillow:
  Thenar eminence wasting? Palmar erythema? Vasculitic lesions?

Feel

• Examine each hand in turn and work distally through the rays of bones (i.e. wrist, MCPs, PIPs, then DIPs).
• Quickly run your hands over the wrist, MCPs, PIPs and DIPs:
  Any increased warmth?
• Support the patient's hands with the tips of your fingers. Roll your thumbs over the dorsum of the wrist and MCPs. Pinch the PIPs and DIPs from the sides. Apply enough pressure to blanch your nail. You must aim to detect tenderness but not hurt the patient!
  Swelling—presence, quality and pattern?
  Joint tenderness?

Move

• Assess wrist extension and flexion actively and passively.
• Assess power and pincer grip.
• Assess hand function, e.g. ask them to hold a pen or pick a coin off the table.

Tips

• Assessment of median and ulnar nerve function is not routinely necessary unless the history is suggestive or there is evidence of thenar or hypothenar wasting
• All examiners or physicians will expect you to recognise and describe the obvious features of rheumatoid arthritis. Additional details to include are assessment of disease activity (based on number of swollen and tender joints) and functional capacity

---

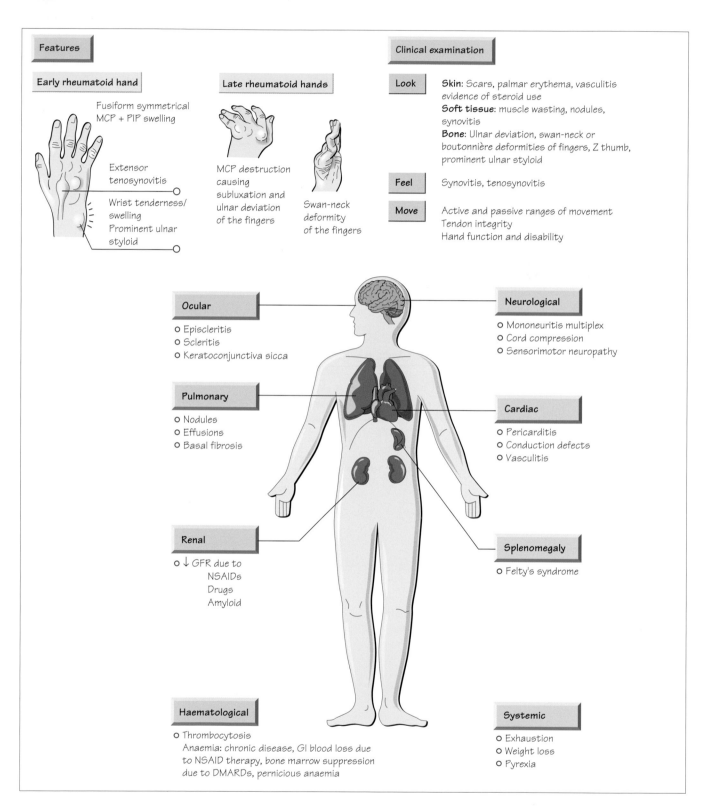

Features

Early rheumatoid hand

Fusiform symmetrical MCP + PIP swelling

Extensor tenosynovitis

Wrist tenderness/ swelling
Prominent ulnar styloid

Late rheumatoid hands

MCP destruction causing subluxation and ulnar deviation of the fingers

Swan-neck deformity of the fingers

Clinical examination

Look

Skin: Scars, palmar erythema, vasculitis evidence of steroid use
Soft tissue: muscle wasting, nodules, synovitis
Bone: Ulnar deviation, swan-neck or boutonnière deformities of fingers, Z thumb, prominent ulnar styloid

Feel Synovitis, tenosynovitis

Move Active and passive ranges of movement
Tendon integrity
Hand function and disability

Ocular
- Episcleritis
- Scleritis
- Keratoconjunctiva sicca

Neurological
- Mononeuritis multiplex
- Cord compression
- Sensorimotor neuropathy

Pulmonary
- Nodules
- Effusions
- Basal fibrosis

Cardiac
- Pericarditis
- Conduction defects
- Vasculitis

Renal
- ↓ GFR due to NSAIDs
  Drugs
  Amyloid

Splenomegaly
- Felty's syndrome

Haematological
- Thrombocytosis
  Anaemia: chronic disease, GI blood loss due to NSAID therapy, bone marrow suppression due to DMARDs, pernicious anaemia

Systemic
- Exhaustion
- Weight loss
- Pyrexia

Introduction

Rheumatoid arthritis (RA) affects 1% of the population and is a leading cause of disability and loss of earnings in a relatively young patient group. In addition, RA increases mortality due to:
- Extra-articular involvement of the renal and respiratory tracts.
- Opportunistic infections in the presence of immunosuppressive drug therapy.
- Accelerated atheroma and subsequent coronary artery disease.

The underlying cause is unknown but is likely to encompass genetic factors, sex hormones and an unidentified initiating agent. B-cells, T-cells and the pro-inflammatory cytokines interleukin 1 (IL-1), IL-6 and tumour necrosis factor α (TNFα) generate persistent cellular activation, autoimmunity and inflammation of synovial joints and of a number of extra-articular sites.

American College of Rheumatology Diagnostic Criteria (1987)

At least four of the following criteria must be met to make a diagnosis of RA. There are no exclusion criteria. Note that joint symptoms must be present for at least 6 weeks to differentiate RA from the post-viral arthropathies (e.g. parvovirus), which generally have a shorter time course and more benign prognosis.

Criteria	Comments
Morning stiffness	Duration > 1 hour (for > 6 weeks)
Arthritis of at least three joints	Soft tissue swelling (for > 6 weeks)
Arthritis of hand joints	MCPs, PIPs or wrist (for > 6 weeks)
Symmetrical arthritis	At least one area (for > 6 weeks)
Rheumatoid nodules	Positive rheumatoid factor
Radiographic changes	Periarticular erosions

Other radiographic features include soft tissue swelling, periarticular osteopaenia, and joint fusion or destruction.

Clinical features

The most common presentation is insidious pain, swelling and stiffness of the small joints of the hands (metacarpophalangeal (MCP) and proximal interphalangeal (PIP) joints, with characteristic sparing of the distal interphalangeals (DIPs)), although any synovial joint may be affected. In contrast to osteoarthritis, the symptoms are most marked in the morning, exacerbated by rest and improve with activity. In a minority of cases the disease can present acutely with widespread synovitis, with a migratory arthritis (palindromic RA) or with marked systemic features of pyrexia, fatigue and weight loss.

As the disease progresses, joint instability leads to subluxation and persistent deformity. Classic changes include:
- Subluxation at the MCP joints with palmar and **ulnar deviation** of the fingers.
- Disease at the PIP joints causes:

  boutonnière deformity (fixed flexion at the PIP and extension at the DIP);

swan-neck deformity (fixed extension at PIP and flexion at DIP);

Z thumb.
- Subluxation and radial deviation at the wrist causing prominence of the ulnar styloid.

Additional musculoskeletal features include:
- (**Stenosing**) **tenosynovitis** causing trigger finger or finger drop if a tendon body is eroded. The extensor digiti minimi is most vulnerable in this regard and the presence of a little finger drop on clinical examination is a warning sign of further tendon damage and profound risk to hand function.
- **Bursitis**.

RA is a systemic disease and its extra-articular features are outlined in the figure opposite.

Treatment

The spectrum of RA requires a multidisciplinary approach involving:
- Specialist nurses – patient education and support, self-care groups.
- Physiotherapy – exercise and joint protection.
- Occupational therapy – adaption, aids and splints.
- Pharmacotherapy – pain and disease control.
- Surgery – joint replacement, arthrodesis and tendon repair.

Pharmacotherapy

RA is treated aggressively as early as possible to prevent deformity and disability and the aim of treatment is total remission.

Non-steroidal anti-inflammatories (NSAIDs)

NSAIDs can be used periodically or continuously. COX-specific inhibitors have a good gastric safety profile but should be avoided in those with heart disease.

Disease-modifying antirheumatic drugs (DMARDs)

DMARDs aim to halt disease progression. Although well tolerated, they have a number of side effects and patients therefore need close monitoring. A patient with difficult disease may often require combinations of two or three DMARDs.

Listed below are the commonest DMARDs, along with their mechanism of action and side effects:
- Methotrexate (folic acid antagonist) + folic acid: myelosuppression, pneumonitis, hepatitis.
- Hydroxychloroquine (inhibition of cellular enzyme release): macular damage.
- Sulphasalazine (mechanism unknown): myelosuppression, rash, hepatitis.
- Leflunomide (arrests activated lymphocytes): myelosuppression, hepatitis, diarrhoea.

Other effective DMARDs include azathioprine, gold, penicillamine, cyclosporin and cyclophosphamide.

Steroids

Systemic steroids are effective in active disease or during flare and can be used to control symptoms until DMARDs have taken effect. High-dose systemic administration is reserved for refractory RA and extra-articular complications not responding to immunotherapy. Intra-articular steroid injections are useful in acute flares; the dramatic beneficial effect is short-lived and has no impact on eventual outcome.

Biological therapy

TNFα blockers are highly effective. Three forms are available:
• Infliximab (chimeric human-murine monoclonal antibody against TNFα).
• Adalimumab (fully humanised monoclonal antibody).
• Etanercept (TNFα:Fc fusion protein.)

TNFα blockade risks opportunistic infection and reactivation of latent TB, and therefore all patients are screened with a chest X-ray and Heaf test prior to biological therapy. The risk and cost of these drugs have given rise to specific NICE (National Institute of Clinical Excellence) guidelines on their use. TNF blockade is restricted to patients with active disease who have failed treatment with at least two DMARDs, of which one must be methotrexate. The clinical improvement only lasts the duration of treatment.

Tips

• Not all patients with rheumatoid arthritis have a positive rheumatoid factor, and not all patients with a positive rheumatoid factor have rheumatoid arthritis
• Disease-modifying antirheumatic drugs (DMARDs) may halt disease progression but will not reverse damage already done
• TNF blockers are effective but carry the risk of susceptibility to infection and reactivation of latent TB

23 The spondyloarthropathies

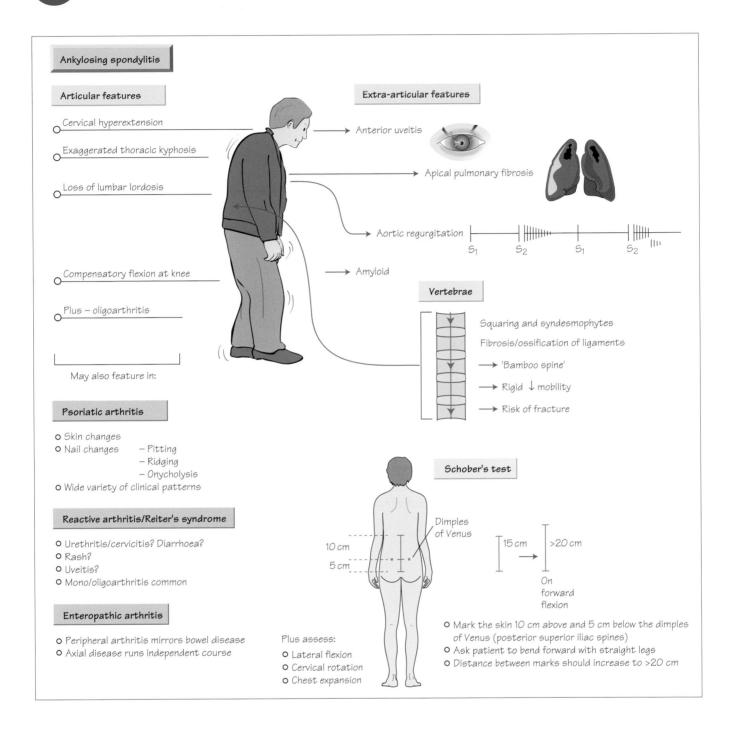

Ankylosing spondylitis

Articular features

- Cervical hyperextension
- Exaggerated thoracic kyphosis
- Loss of lumbar lordosis
- Compensatory flexion at knee
- Plus – oligoarthritis

May also feature in:

Psoriatic arthritis

- Skin changes
- Nail changes — Pitting
  — Ridging
  — Onycholysis
- Wide variety of clinical patterns

Reactive arthritis/Reiter's syndrome

- Urethritis/cervicitis? Diarrhoea?
- Rash?
- Uveitis?
- Mono/oligoarthritis common

Enteropathic arthritis

- Peripheral arthritis mirrors bowel disease
- Axial disease runs independent course

Extra-articular features

- Anterior uveitis
- Apical pulmonary fibrosis
- Aortic regurgitation

  S_1 S_2 S_1 S_2

- Amyloid

Vertebrae

Squaring and syndesmophytes
Fibrosis/ossification of ligaments
→ 'Bamboo spine'
→ Rigid ↓ mobility
→ Risk of fracture

Schober's test

10 cm
5 cm
Dimples of Venus

15 cm → >20 cm
On forward flexion

- Mark the skin 10 cm above and 5 cm below the dimples of Venus (posterior superior iliac spines)
- Ask patient to bend forward with straight legs
- Distance between marks should increase to >20 cm

Plus assess:
- Lateral flexion
- Cervical rotation
- Chest expansion

Introduction

Spondyloarthropathies is a collective term for a group of inflammatory joint diseases that may involve the spine. The classic spondyloarthropathy is **ankylosing spondylitis** in which pelvic and axial disease is the predominant feature, but inflammatory spinal disease may also occur in **psoriatic**, **reactive** or **enteropathic arthritis**. The spondyloarthropathies share a number of features that may affect an individual patient at any time during the course of their disease:

- Sacroiliac/pelviaxial disease (back or buttock pain).
- Peripheral inflammatory arthropathy (any pattern of joint disease).
- Enthesopathy (inflammation of tendon insertions, classically Achilles).
- Non-musculoskeletal syndromes (e.g. skin or eye disease).

In addition, the spondyloarthropathies share an association with the MHC molecule HLA-B27, and the closeness of this association varies with the clinical subtype. For example, more than

90% of patients with ankylosing spondylitis (AS) are HLA-B27 positive compared with 50% of those with psoriatic or enteropathic arthritis.

Ankylosing spondylitis

AS classically presents with insidious inflammatory back pain and morning stiffness that improves with activity and deteriorates with rest. Typically the patients are young (< 40 years) and male (ratio 3 male : 1 female), and a family history of spinal disease may be available.

Symptoms are caused by fibrosis and ossification of ligaments, tendons and insertions, mainly in the region of the intervertebral discs and the sacroiliac joints, and eventually spinal fusion may occur as a result of syndesmophyte formation (bridging spurs of bone at the corner of adjacent vertebral bodies). Spinal fusion is surprisingly painless until microfractures occur.

Chest expansion is reduced by disease at the costovertebral and costochondral junctions.

Insertional tendonitis and peripheral synovitis (mono- or oligoarticular) occur in a significant proportion of patients.

Advanced AS produces a **'question-mark' posture**, characterised by:
- loss of lumbar lordosis;
- exaggerated thoracic kyphosis;
- cervical hyperextension;
- compensatory flexion at the knee.

Clinical assessment of AS relies on assessment of chest expansion and spinal mobility, by measuring both lateral and forward flexion (**Schober's test**, see opposite).

AS has a number of *extra-articular associations*:
- Anterior uveitis occurs in up to 40% of patients with AS, but its occurrence bears no relation to disease activity in the spine.
- Apical pulmonary fibrosis, pleuritis and fusion of thoracic chest wall cause restrictive lung disease and all patients must be advised against smoking.
- Aortic incompetence.

Diagnosis

Diagnosis hinges on a combination of radiological evidence of sacroiliitis and either a typical history or examination findings. Additional radiological features in AS include:
- squaring of vertebrae;
- ossification;
- syndesmophytes;
- facet joint involvement.

Treatment

The mainstay of therapy is patient education, physiotherapy and non-steroidal anti-inflammatory drugs (NSAIDs) for spinal disease. Peripheral disease may be controlled by sulphasalazine.

Psoriatic arthritis

Five to 10% of patients with psoriasis develop arthritis. The male: female ratio is equivalent, with a peak incidence between 20 and 40 years of age. Clinical patterns vary widely including:
- distal hand disease predominantly affecting the distal interphalangeal (DIP) joints;

- symmetrical polyarthritis similar to rheumatoid arthritis;
- spondyloarthropathy;
- asymmetrical oligoarthritis;
- arthritis mutilans due to osteolysis of the small joints in the hand.

Dactylitis (so-called 'sausage finger'), tenosynovitis and enthesitis are also common.

Diagnosis

Differentiating rheumatoid arthritis (RA) in a patient with coexistent psoriasis from true psoriatic arthritis (PsA) can be difficult, especially since up to 10% of those with PsA are rheumatoid factor positive. However, the presence of disease at the DIP joint and/or psoriatic nail changes (pitting, ridging, onycholysis, salmon-pink patches) would suggest an underlying diagnosis of PsA rather than RA. Radiological indicators of a diagnosis of PsA rather than RA include:
- Absence of juxta-articular osteopaenia.
- Whittling of the terminal phalanges (acro-osteolysis).
- Pencil-in-cup deformity (erosion of the proximal and expansion of the distal portion of an interphalangeal joint).
- Ankylosis.

Since psoriasis is a high cell turnover state, hyperuricaemia and gout are also possible causes for arthropathy in this population.

Treatment

- NSAIDs and occasional intra-articular steroid injection can be used as a 'rescue'.
- Methotrexate and/or leflunomide (may also improve skin).
- Sulphasalazine, azathioprine, penicillamine, gold and cyclosporin in severe cases.
- Avoid use of hydroxychloroquine as it may produce flares of skin disease.

Reactive arthritis/Reiter's syndrome

Any of the spondyloarthropathies are considered 'reactive' if a history of urethritis/cervicitis or diarrhoea is present. Urethritis is commonly due to *Chlamydia* and may be asymptomatic; the diarrhoeal illness has usually occurred within the preceding month and the most likely pathogens are *Shigella*, *Salmonella* and *Campylobacter*. The syndrome may develop acutely with fever, weight loss and polyarticular involvement, but more commonly patients present with a mono- or oligoarthritis and either a low grade or absent fever.

Additional features that may be present include:
- Balanitis circinata: painless plaques on the glans or shaft of the penis.
- Keratoderma blennorrhagica: a painless papular/pustular rash on the palms or soles of the feet.
- Conjunctivitis: may be followed by uveitis.

Recurrent/repeated infections do not always lead to recurrence of arthritis. Other post-infective arthropathy differentials include HIV, Lyme disease, Behçet's disease and parvovirus.

Diagnosis

The diagnosis relies on a careful history/examination and the combination of raised inflammatory markers, as well as the results of serologic testing, cultures and swabs. Joint aspirate will rule out a septic or crystal arthropathy. There are no classic radiological features.

Treatment

NSAIDs and local corticosteroid injections will suffice for many patients, and the majority are in remission within 2 years. However, persistent disease may require DMARDs such as sulphasalazine.

Antibiotic therapy against the precipitating infection may not have any impact on the arthropathy.

Enteric arthropathy

Up to 20% of patients with either Crohn's disease or ulcerative colitis develop an arthropathy.

• **Peripheral disease** (mono- or oligoarthritis, most commonly knee or ankle) has a higher incidence in Crohn's patients. It may coincide with the onset of bowel disease and has a close association between exacerbations.
• **Sacroiliitis** occurs in both forms of inflammatory bowel disease.

It is not clearly associated with either the onset or exacerbations of bowel pathology.

Treatment

Therapy relies on NSAIDs, intra-articular and/or oral steroids and sulphasalazine if disease-modifying therapy is required.

Tips

• Virtually all patients with ankylosing spondylitis are HLA-B27 positive, but not all HLA-B27 patients have ankylosing spondylitis
• Nail changes are a characteristic feature of those with psoriatic arthritis
• Most patients with reactive arthritis are in remission within 2 years
• Spinal and bowel disease run independent courses in enteric arthropathy

---

Acute joint disease

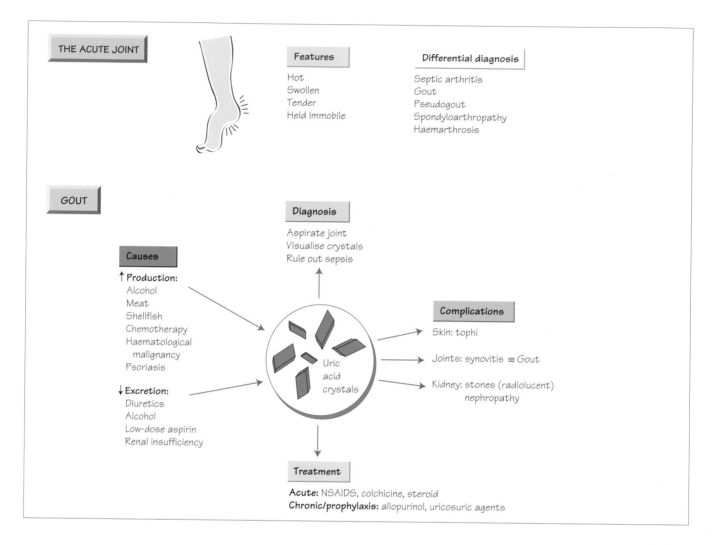

THE ACUTE JOINT

Features

Hot
Swollen
Tender
Held immobile

Differential diagnosis

Septic arthritis
Gout
Pseudogout
Spondyloarthropathy
Haemarthrosis

GOUT

Diagnosis

Aspirate joint
Visualise crystals
Rule out sepsis

Causes

↑ Production:
Alcohol
Meat
Shellfish
Chemotherapy
Haematological
  malignancy
Psoriasis

↓ Excretion:
Diuretics
Alcohol
Low-dose aspirin
Renal insufficiency

Uric acid crystals

Complications

Skin: tophi

Joints: synovitis ≡ Gout

Kidney: stones (radiolucent)
  nephropathy

Treatment

Acute: NSAIDS, colchicine, steroid
Chronic/prophylaxis: allopurinol, uricosuric agents

Introduction

An acutely painful, swollen or hot joint is a medical emergency. It is crucial to rule out septic arthritis, but one of the most common causes is an acute crystal arthropathy, i.e. **gout** or **pseudogout**.

Gout

Gout is an inflammatory arthropathy generated by uric acid crystal deposition in the joints and peri-articular structures, e.g. bursae. Uric acid is a product of DNA breakdown (purine nucleotides) but is also present in foods and alcohol. Once a biochemical threshold is reached in a susceptible individual, crystals precipitate into joints, skin and kidneys causing a spectrum of disease.

Clinical picture

Gout is characterised by acute attacks of joint inflammation separated by asymptomatic periods. The commonest joint to be affected is the first metatarsophalangeal joint (**podagra**), but other common sites include the ankle, knee, wrist and fingers. Attacks are usually monoarticular but may become polyarticular

if recurrent attacks are left untreated, and indeed this chronic inflammation can generate a destructive arthritis.

Hyperuricaemia can be generated by two processes.

1 Overproduction of urate or increased purine synthesis. A number of different things can cause this overproduction:
   • Alcohol, red meats and seafood contain high levels of urate.
   • Increased cell turnover states such as psoriasis, haematological malignancies or chemotherapy produce purines via DNA breakdown.
   • Enzyme defects can also be responsible, but these are relatively rare.

2 Underexcretion of urate. This can be due to renal failure, alcohol, diuretics, low dose aspirin, dehydration or starvation.

Frequently an attack of gout is provoked by trauma, surgery or alcohol/dietary excess.

Note that biochemical hyperuricaemia may not produce the clinical syndrome of gout.

Uric acid deposition in the skin produces **tophi** – well demarcated collections of crystals that may rupture, releasing a chalk-like substance. Classic sites for tophi include the helix of the ear, the olecranon and prepatellar bursae, the ulnar border of the forearm and the tendons. Tophi may break down or ulcerate and occasionally cause diagnostic confusion with rheumatoid nodulosis.

Deposition of urate in the renal tract can cause:
• Renal stones (remember that uric acid stones are radiolucent).
• Urate nephropathy (deposition of urate in renal interstitium or collecting tubules).
Thus, gout can both cause and be caused by renal impairment.

Investigations

Urate levels
These may be normal (or even fall) during an acute attack in up to 50% of patients. They are used principally to monitor the success or compliance of urate-lowering therapy.

X-ray
X-rays show soft tissue swelling, and punched-out erosions in persistent disease which may corticate and heal. Osteopaenia is not a feature and joint fusion is rare.

Joint fluid
Joint fluid shows low viscosity, a high white cell count and the presence of intraneutrophilic urate crystals – characteristically needle-shaped and negatively birefringent under polarised microscopy.

Management

Acute attack
The priority is to relieve pain and inflammation using non-steroidal anti-inflammatory agents (NSAIDs), colchicine or steroids.

Prophylaxis
Lifestyle modification (avoidance of risk factors) should be undertaken. Urate-lowering therapy is commenced under anti-inflammatory cover once the acute attack has settled. Allopurinol (xanthine oxidase inhibitor) is used most commonly. Uricosuric agents (increase urate renal excretion) such as probenicid, sulphinpyrazone or benzbromazone are second-line agents, but cannot be used in the presence of renal stones.

Pseudogout
Pseudogout is an inflammatory arthropathy due to calcium pyrophosphate deposition, and is frequently associated with chondrocalcinosis (calcification of fibrocartilage and hyaline cartilage). The commonest presentation is an acutely hot, swollen and tender joint, usually the knee or shoulder, but it can present more insidiously as a 'pseudorheumatoid' polyarticular pattern in the hand. Underlying disease states (including haemachromatosis, Wilson's disease and hyperparathyroidism) may precipitate pseudogout and these should be sought in a young patient with this diagnosis.

Diagnosis relies on the identification of positively birefringent rhomboid-shaped crystals in synovial fluid.

NSAIDs are the mainstay of treatment, in combination with joint aspiration and intra-articular steroid injection. Low-dose colchicine may play a role in prophylaxis.

Differential diagnosis of the acute joint
1 An acute joint is **septic arthritis** until proven otherwise. Although septic arthritis is *not* the most common final diagnosis, it must be considered in all cases, including those with established inflammatory arthropathy, as its consequences are dire.
2 Crystal arthropathy (see above).
3 Flare of established **inflammatory arthropathy**, e.g. rheumatoid, psoriatic or enteric arthropathy, or Reiter's syndrome.
4 Intra-articular bleed (haemarthrosis) in patients with bleeding diathesis or on warfarin therapy.

It should also be remembered that inflammation in periarticular structures (e.g. bursitis or tendinopathy) can mimic a hot joint. Ultrasound investigation can prove very helpful in these situations.

Summary
If a patient presents with an acutely inflamed joint, you are obliged to rule out septic arthritis. Crystal arthropathy or a seronegative spondyloarthropathy are also possible culprits. There are a number of features one should elicit in the history to determine the most likely underlying diagnosis:
• Is the patient *septic*?
• Risk factors/history of *gout*?
• Known inflammatory arthropathy, e.g. *spondylarthritis*?
• Rash? *Psoriatic arthropathy/Reiter's syndrome/enteric arthropathy*.
• Diarrhoea? *Reiter's syndrome/enteric arthropathy*.
• Eye disease? *Reiter's syndrome/enteric arthropathy*.
• Known sexually transmitted disease or urethral discharge? *Reiter's syndrome*.
• Warfarin or bleeding episodes? *Haemarthrosis*.

The single most important investigation is **synovial fluid aspiration**. The fluid must be sent immediately for microscopy, culture and sensitivity studies to rule out septic arthritis or crystal arthropathy.

Tips
• An acute monoarthritis is septic arthritis until proven otherwise – and joint aspiration is mandatory
• Gout would be unusual in a premenopausal woman
• Urate levels may be normal during an acute attack of gout

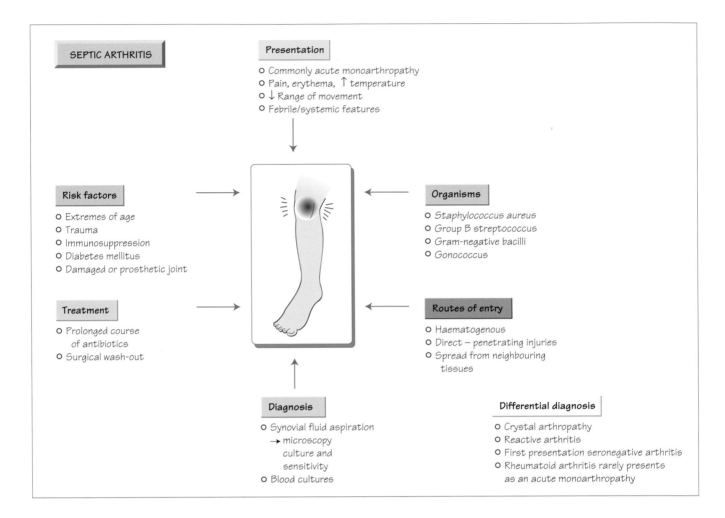

SEPTIC ARTHRITIS

Presentation
- o Commonly acute monoarthropathy
- o Pain, erythema, ↑ temperature
- o ↓ Range of movement
- o Febrile/systemic features

Risk factors
- o Extremes of age
- o Trauma
- o Immunosuppression
- o Diabetes mellitus
- o Damaged or prosthetic joint

Treatment
- o Prolonged course of antibiotics
- o Surgical wash-out

Organisms
- o *Staphylococcus aureus*
- o Group B streptococcus
- o Gram-negative bacilli
- o Gonococcus

Routes of entry
- o Haematogenous
- o Direct – penetrating injuries
- o Spread from neighbouring tissues

Diagnosis
- o Synovial fluid aspiration
  → microscopy culture and sensitivity
- o Blood cultures

Differential diagnosis
- o Crystal arthropathy
- o Reactive arthritis
- o First presentation seronegative arthritis
- o Rheumatoid arthritis rarely presents as an acute monoarthropathy

Septic arthritis

Septic arthritis is a rheumatological emergency. It is associated with considerable morbidity and mortality (up to 15%), so a high index of suspicion should always be maintained.

Clinical features

A septic joint is exquisitely painful and is often held rigid in the most comfortable position. Systemic features of infection such as fever and constitutional upset are typical but occasionally patients may be afebrile and appear deceptively well. Although the classic presentation of bacterial arthritis is an acute mono-arthritis, up to a third of cases are polyarticular.

Patients at particular risk of developing septic arthritis include:
- Patients with abnormal, damaged or prosthetic joints.
- The immunocompromised (including diabetics).
- The elderly and the very young.

Bacteria reach the joint through three major routes:
1 Haematogenous spread during an episode of bacteraemia.
2 Direct inoculation following a penetrating injury, surgery or joint injection.

3 Spread from neighbouring bone (osteomyelitis) or soft tissue (cellulitis).

Diagnosis

The diagnosis hinges on joint aspiration and analysis of the synovial fluid. In non-gonococcal bacterial arthritis, the yield from joint cultures is > 95%, falling to 50% yield from blood cultures. In high-risk or clear-cut cases it is prudent to commence antibiotic therapy as soon as joint fluid and blood cultures have been taken; antimicrobial therapy can be adjusted once the microbiological results and sensitivities are available.

The commonest **causative agents** are divided into:
1 Non-gonococcal (80% cases):
- *Staphylococcus aureus*;
- B haemolytic streptococci;
- Gram-negative bacilli, e.g. *Pseudomonas*, *Escherichia coli* and *Proteus*.

In children, *Streptococcus* and *Haemophilus influenzae* are the commonest pathogens.
2 Gonococcal arthritis.

Occasionally gonococcal arthritis can be clinically differentiated from non-gonococcal disease and this can prevent considerable diagnostic delay – microbiological yield in gonococcal disease is notoriously poor with up to 75% of synovial fluid cultures being negative. In addition, positive blood cultures are exceedingly rare. Gonococcal septic arthritis tends to occur in younger, healthier patients, the arthritis may adopt a migratory pattern and tenosynovitis and skin lesions are a frequent feature. It is important to remember that the antecedent infection may be asymptomatic, particularly in women.

Treatment

The treatment of choice for septic arthritis is appropriate **antibiotic therapy** – empiric choices *must* cover staphylococcal and streptococcal species and most patients receive 6 weeks of antibiotics. Surgical wash-out of a joint (especially prosthetic ones) may be warranted.

Osteomyelitis

Osteomyelitis is infection of bone or bone marrow and usually presents with deep-seated bone pain, with or without septic features. The majority of cases in adults are caused by *Staphylococcus aureus*, but tuberculosis, salmonella and pseudomonas are also encountered.

Diagnosis

Diagnosis relies on appropriate imaging. The earliest changes of marrow oedema can be visualised on MRI, whereas CT is better at demonstrating the development of vascular congestion or thrombosis. The 'classic' periosteal reaction is seen late in disease, e.g. at 2–3 weeks, but is evident on a plain radiograph. Remember that the white cell count and inflammatory response may be normal despite active infection.

Treatment

Treatment is similar to that for the infected joint, with prolonged courses of appropriate antibiotics. Occasionally, surgical debridement is required.

Malignant bone tumours

Secondary tumours are far more common than primary bone malignancy. The commonest carcinomas to spread to bone are breast, bronchus, thyroid, prostate and kidney and the commonest sites for deposit are the vertebral column, ribs, proximal femur and humerus.
• Metastatic deposits tend to erode bone (**lytic lesions**) and may present with vertebral collapse or pathological fracture.

Extensive destruction may cause **hypercalcaemia**, but more frequently the hypercalcaemia of malignancy is due to the production of parathyroid hormone-related protein by tumour cells.
• Prostate and occasionally breast secondaries may induce reactive new bone formation, giving rise to **osteosclerotic metastases**. These patients will have a high serum **alkaline phosphatase**.
• Bone pain from malignancy is unremitting. **Night pain** is a classic 'red flag' symptom for malignancy.
• Treatment centres on management of the hypercalcaemia, surgical stabilisation of deposits at risk of fracture, radiotherapy and pain control.

The commonest primary malignant diseases of bone are **myeloma** and **osteosarcoma**.

Myeloma

• Multiple myeloma is caused by neoplastic proliferation of plasma cells in the bone marrow leading to bone pain and pathological fractures. If the marrow is replaced by tumour cells a **pancytopaenia** may result.
• Radiologically, myeloma causes multiple '**punched-out**' lesions; if the disease is widespread a diffuse **osteoporosis** may occur.
• Classically myeloma patients have a high erythrocyte sedimentation rate (ESR), elevated calcium and alkaline phosphatase, a monoclonal protein in the serum (and urine) and typical cellular changes in the marrow.

Osteosarcoma

• Osteosarcoma affects young people, with most cases occurring between 10 and 25 years of age.
• Patients typically present with pain and swelling but pathological fracture is relatively unusual.
• The majority of osteosarcomas arise in the metaphysis of the long bones. Classic sites include the knee, proximal humerus and femur and distal radius.
• Treatment involves chemotherapy and surgery.

Tips

• Any patient presenting with an acute monoarthritis should be assumed to have septic arthritis until proven otherwise
• Never inject a joint through infected skin or soft tissues
• Think of myeloma in an elderly patient with osteoporosis and/or fracture in the presence of an unexplained elevated ESR

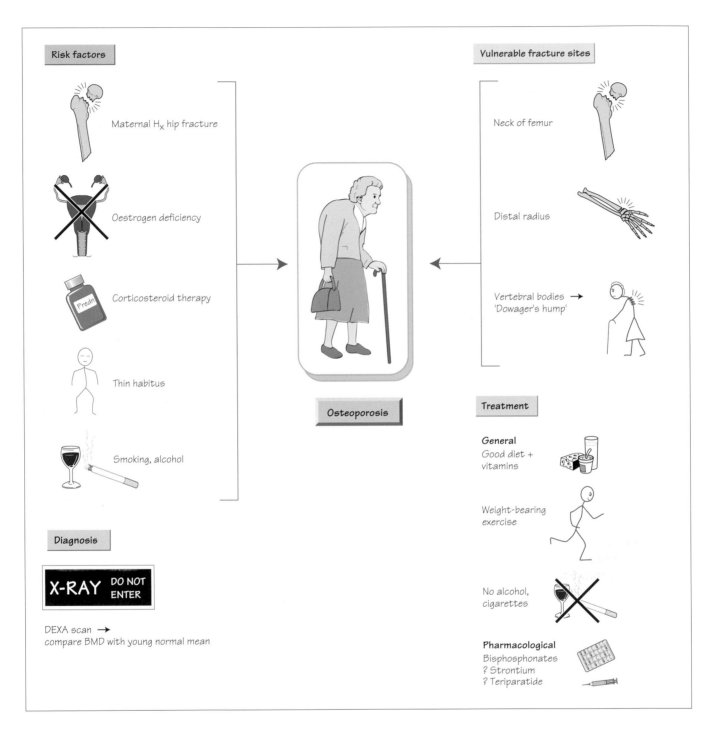

Introduction

The World Health Organisation has defined osteoporosis as a 'systemic skeletal disease characterised by low bone mass and microarchitectural deterioration of bone tissue with a consequent increase in bone fragility and susceptibility to fracture'. **Bone mass** or mineral density relies on a balance between osteoblastic and osteoclastic activity. Overall bone mass increases until adulthood, plateaus and then declines from 35 years of age onwards, accelerating in women following the menopause.

By 60–70 years of age, 30% of women have osteoporosis, rising to 70% in those over 80 years. Although the entire skeleton is affected, the commonest sites for **osteoporotic fracture** are the neck of the femur, the vertebrae and the distal radius. The morbidity associated with neck of femur fractures is particularly significant, and generates an increasing economic burden.

Risk factors

The most important risk factors for osteoporosis are:

- Maternal family history of hip fracture.
- Oestrogen deficiency, e.g. due to premature menopause, prolonged secondary amenorrhoea or primary hypogonadism.
- Corticosteroid therapy, e.g. prednisolone dose > 7.5 mg/day for > 6 months.
- Low body mass index (BMI) of < 19 kg/m^2) due to a combination of reduced oestrogen levels and reduction in impact loading.
  Other risk factors include:
- Smoking.
- Excess alcohol.
- Anorexia nervosa (low weight, menstrual irregularity, low calcium intake).
- Endocrine syndromes (hyperparathyroidism, hyperthyroidism, Cushing's syndrome).
- Inflammatory arthropathy (probably due to increased IL-1 and TNFα levels).
- Prolonged immobilisation.

Diagnosis

Osteoporosis is diagnosed using a dual energy X-ray absorptiometry or DEXA scan. This allows a measurement of the **bone mineral density** (BMD) at the lumbar spine and proximal femur for comparison with that of the young normal mean – the T score.

- **Normal**: BMD > 1 standard deviation (SD) *below* the young normal mean (more than −1).
- **Osteopaenia**: BMD 1–2.5 SD *below* the young normal mean (between −1 and −2.5).
- **Osteoporosis**: BMD > 2.5 SD *below* the young normal mean (more than −2.5).
- **Severe osteoporosis**: as above plus previous fragility fracture.

Treatment

General measures

All patients with osteoporosis must maintain good nutrition with high levels of calcium and vitamin D, by dietary supplementation if necessary. Increased physical activity improves BMD via impact loading and also reduces the overall risk of falls. Patients should also be advised to stop smoking and to avoid alcohol excess, and steroid doses must be reduced or withdrawn wherever possible.

Pharmacological measures

Bisphosphonates: risedronate, alendronate, etidronate

As a group, the bisphosphonates inhibit the action and function of osteoclasts, thereby reducing skeletal resorption and the subsequent risk of fracture at both vertebral and non-vertebral sites. They are available as daily or weekly preparations, but have variable acceptability and compliance due to gastrointestinal side effects. In order to reduce side effects and to maximise otherwise relatively poor absorption, patients must take their bisphosphonate on an empty stomach, with plenty of water, remain upright for 30 minutes after ingestion and have nothing to eat or drink for a further 30 minutes.

Selective oestrogen receptor modulators (SERMs): raloxifene

SERMs such as raloxifene have oestrogenic effects on bone, but not breast or endometrium. They have been shown to decrease bone turnover in post-menopausal women with a subsequent increase in BMD and a reduction in vertebral (but not hip) fracture rate. In general they are well-tolerated, but confer an increased risk of deep venous thrombosis.

Strontium

Although its precise mechanism of action is unclear, strontium appears to uncouple bone remodelling, thereby stimulating bone formation and increasing BMD at the lumbar spine and femoral neck. It has a proven role in reducing vertebral fracture rate and preliminary data from a large clinical trial also suggest a reduction in hip fracture risk.

Teriparatide (synthetic parathyroid hormone)

Exogenous parathyroid hormone has been shown to have anabolic effects on bone, increasing BMD and reducing the osteoporotic fracture rate. Currently licensed for the treatment of severe osteoporosis, it is administered as a once-daily subcutaneous injection. However, treatment is limited to 18 months as toxicology studies have suggested an increased risk of osteosarcoma with prolonged use.

Hormone replacement therapy (HRT)

Although it has been shown to increase BMD and reduce fracture rate, HRT should no longer be prescribed for *primary prevention* of osteoporosis as the associated risks of venous thromboembolism and breast carcinoma are deemed unacceptably high. The only current indication for HRT is the management of **menopausal symptoms**; bone protection is simply an additional benefit. **Testosterone** is used in men when hypogonadism is the underlying aetiology of their osteoporosis.

Corticosteroid-induced osteoporosis

Steroid therapy suppresses bone formation, increases osteoblast apoptosis and disrupts calcium homeostasis. For a given BMD, osteoporosis caused by steroids has the highest rate of fracture. There is a strong correlation between the daily dose and the fracture risk, and the risk both increases and declines rapidly on and off treatment. All physicians must be alert to the profound risk of long-term steroid therapy – particularly in the elderly population. The diagnosis and treatment for corticosteroid-induced osteoporosis is identical to that for idiopathic disease.

> ### Tips
>
> - Consider the diagnosis of osteoporosis in any patient with low trauma fracture
> - Any elderly patient on steroids should receive bone protection
> - Bisphosphonates in combination with vitamin D/calcium supplementation are the first-line treatment in primary and secondary prevention of osteoporosis

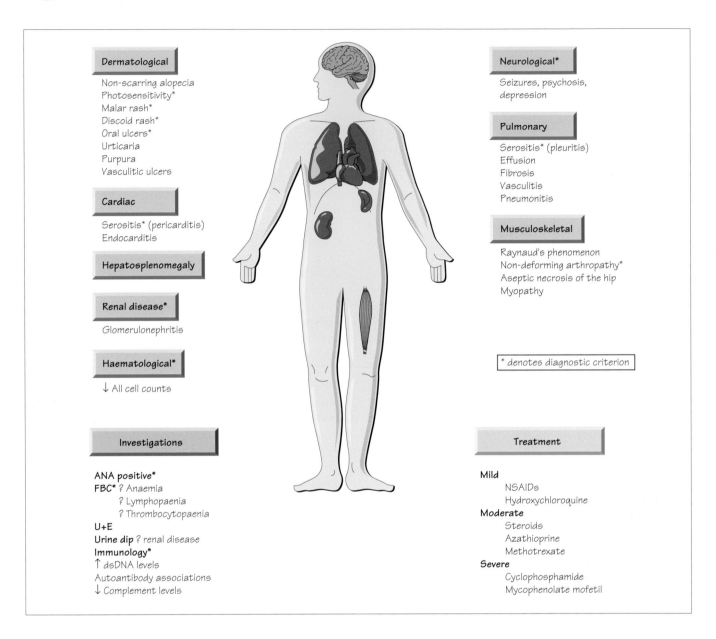

Dermatological

Non-scarring alopecia
Photosensitivity*
Malar rash*
Discoid rash*
Oral ulcers*
Urticaria
Purpura
Vasculitic ulcers

Cardiac

Serositis* (pericarditis)
Endocarditis

Hepatosplenomegaly

Renal disease*

Glomerulonephritis

Haematological*

↓ All cell counts

Investigations

ANA positive*
FBC* ? Anaemia
      ? Lymphopaenia
      ? Thrombocytopaenia
U+E
Urine dip ? renal disease
Immunology*
↑ dsDNA levels
Autoantibody associations
↓ Complement levels

Neurological*

Seizures, psychosis,
depression

Pulmonary

Serositis* (pleuritis)
Effusion
Fibrosis
Vasculitis
Pneumonitis

Musculoskeletal

Raynaud's phenomenon
Non-deforming arthropathy*
Aseptic necrosis of the hip
Myopathy

* denotes diagnostic criterion

Treatment

Mild
    NSAIDs
    Hydroxychloroquine
Moderate
    Steroids
    Azathioprine
    Methotrexate
Severe
    Cyclophosphamide
    Mycophenolate mofetil

Introduction

Systemic lupus erythematosus (SLE) is a complex, multisystem, autoimmune condition characterised by autoantibodies directed against nuclear components. The variety of autoantigens (e.g. histone, ribonucleoprotein (RNP)) is responsible for an array of patterns and severity of disease, which can range from mild to life-threatening in the same patient over time. The variable and multisystem nature of SLE makes it a great mimic of other conditions, and it can be a difficult diagnosis to make. As a result, clinicians have adopted the diagnostic criteria of the American Rheumatological Association (ARA), which were originally created for research and epidemiological purposes.

ARA diagnostic criteria for SLE

Four or more of the following must be fulfilled, either simultaneously or sequentially.

Malar 'butterfly' rash	Non-scarring rash over cheeks and bridge of nose
Discoid rash	Scarring rash commonly in sun-exposed areas
Photosensitivity	
Oral ulcers	
Arthralgia	Non-erosive arthropathy
Serositis	Pleuritis, pericarditis
Renal disease	Proteinuria > 0.5 g per 24 hours or cellular casts
Haematological	Haemolytic anaemia, leucopaenia or lymphopaenia
Neurological	Seizures, psychosis
Antinuclear antibody (ANA)	Raised ANA titre
Immunological disorder	Raised dsDNA or anti-Sm antibody titres Positive antiphospholipid antibodies

Skin disease and arthropathy

In addition to the skin symptoms in the diagnostic criteria, patients with cutaneous manifestations of lupus may present with non-scarring alopecia, purpura, urticaria and hyperpigmentation. The musculoskeletal picture is dominated by **polyarticular arthralgia**, but the disease is more benign than rheumatoid arthritis and overt joint damage occurs in fewer than 10% of patients. **Jaccoud's arthropathy** refers to reversible joint instability and subluxation due to tendonitis rather than irreversible destruction due to synovitis. Muscle disease is rare and may be a consequence of drug therapy.

Renal lupus

Renal disease is a serious complication and every patient should have their blood pressure checked, electrolytes measured and urine assessed for casts and protein at each clinic visit. SLE causes a range of glomerulonephritidies, which have been classified by the World Health Organisation according to biopsy findings. Although this system may offer some clues to prognosis, renal lupus is generally treated very aggressively.

Respiratory disease

Up to two-thirds of patients will complain of pain or **pleuritis** at some point during their disease, and a third develop pleural effusions. The more unusual complications of interstitial fibrosis, vasculitis and pneumonitis may present with an insidious development of shortness of breath and/or decrease in exercise tolerance. First-line investigations include a chest X-ray and lung function tests, which may indicate a greater extent of disease than is evident clinically. Pulmonary hypertension may occur as a result of fibrosis, vasculopathy or chronic thromboembolic disease, particularly in those with antiphospholipid syndrome (see below).

Haematological system

Autoantibodies against red cells, lymphocytes and platelets may reduce all of these cell counts, and an acute **thrombocytopaenia** can be dramatic and life-threatening. The commonest haematological finding, however, is **anaemia of chronic disease**, which is present in up to three-quarters of lupus patients. While the ESR is commonly raised in SLE, an elevated CRP (C-reactive protein) is unusual and should prompt a search for concurrent infection.

Raynaud's phenomenon

Although not a diagnostic criterion, Raynaud's is common in lupus patients and may predate the disease by some years. Treatment is identical to idiopathic Raynaud's disease with vasodilators.

Drug-induced lupus

Hydralazine, procainamide, isoniazid, minocycline and sulphasalazine have all been implicated in causing SLE, but drug-induced disease is generally mild, with few renal or neurological features and the disease disappears with cessation of the drug.

These medications are not contraindicated in idiopathic SLE.

Serology
Autoantibodies

Autoantibodies directed against the nucleus are *not* specific for lupus but they are very sensitive and therefore a **raised ANA titre** is a useful first step in the diagnosis of SLE. A negative ANA in a patient with suspected SLE is very reassuring, but a raised ANA titre does not always lead to a diagnosis of lupus as elevated levels can be found in a number of other autoimmune conditions such as rheumatoid arthritis or Sjögren's syndrome.

Antibodies directed against native DNA (dsDNA) are more specific for a diagnosis of SLE and the remaining autoantibodies are associated with particular complications as listed below.

Antibody	Prevalence	Association
ANA	> 90%	Not specific, but a diagnostic criterion
DsDNA	40–90%	Renal disease
Histone	30–80%	Drug-induced lupus
Sm	30–80%	SLE-specific if found in Afro-Caribbean patient
RNP	20–35%	Renal disease
Ro	25–40%	Sjögren's syndrome, cutaneous lupus, congenital heart block
La	10–15%	As for Ro

Complement

SLE causes reduced levels of C3 and C4 due to immune complex deposition. In an exacerbation of lupus, the complement levels would be expected to fall, in association with an elevation in dsDNA titre. However, since patients often have persistently abnormal serology in the absence of active disease, results must be assessed in combination with the clinical picture.

Treatment

All lupus patients should avoid sun exposure and use high-factor sun creams. Other treatment varies depending on the severity of the disease.

• **Mild disease**. Non-steroidal anti-inflammatory drugs (NSAIDs) are appropriate for intermittent arthralgia, and hydroxychloroquine is excellent for skin and musculoskeletal disease.

• **Moderate disease**. More persistent disease activity or the presence of haematological features would require the use of oral or pulsed intravenous steroids. Azathioprine or methotrexate can be used as steroid-sparing agents once the disease is under control.

• **Severe disease**. Cyclophosphamide and mycophenolate mofetil are reserved for more serious disease, including renal involvement.

Antiphospholipid syndrome

Antiphospholipid syndrome is a procoagulant state which may occur as a primary phenomenon, or in association with SLE. Symptoms include:

• venous and arterial thrombosis;
• recurrent miscarriage;
• livedo reticularis;
• thrombocytopaenia.

The diagnosis is confirmed by the combination of the clinical picture and the presence of anticardiolipin antibody or lupus anticoagulant (or both). Treatment is anticoagulation.

Tips

• Not all patients with a positive antinuclear factor have SLE
• SLE has a wide range of clinical presentations and severity of disease
• Renal lupus is the most feared complication and should be identified and treated promptly

---

Giant cell arteritis

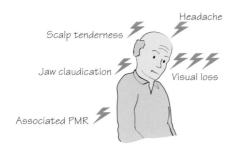

Headache

Scalp tenderness

Jaw claudication

Visual loss

Associated PMR

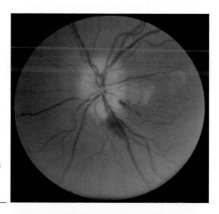

Acute ischaemic optic neuropathy. The optic nerve head (disc) in the affected eye is swollen and pale as the nerve fibres are infarcted. Because this is an arterial ischaemic phenomenon, recovery of nerve function is rare, and optic atrophy supervenes.
Courtesy of Dr Peggy Frith, Oxford Eye Hospital

Investigations

ESR and CRP raised
Temporal artery biopsy
Beware: skip lesions!

Giant cell arteritis.
Temporal artery biopsy shows a narrow lumen and swollen arterial wall. There are widespread inflammatory cells throughout the layers of the artery and several multinucleated 'giant cells' within the media.
Courtesy of Dr Peggy Frith, Oxford Eye Hospital

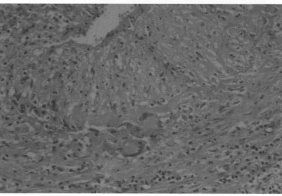

Classification of arteritis

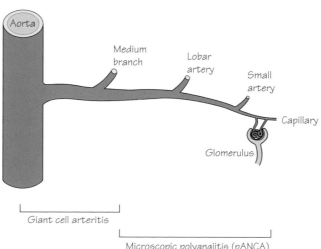

Aorta

Medium branch

Lobar artery

Small artery

Capillary

Glomerulus

Giant cell arteritis

Microscopic polyangiitis (pANCA)
Wegener's granulomatosis (cANCA)
Churg–Strauss

PAN
(ANCA negative)

Introduction

The vasculitidies are a heterogenous group of disorders caused by **vascular inflammation**. As the vessel wall dies, ischaemia and infarction occur distal to the area of necrosis. The easiest system for classifying this group of conditions is therefore by **vessel size**, which aids in prediction of outcome and/or complications. The small vessel vasculitidies are further subdivided according to their association with antineutrophil cytoplasmic antibodies (ANCAs).

1 *Large vessel* (aorta and largest branches): claudication, loss of pulses, cardiac failure, organ infarction.
2 *Medium vessel* (medium-sized arteries and smaller vessels): renal failure, hypertension, purpura.
3 *Small vessel*: renal and skin disease, pulmonary haemorrhage, arthralgia.

The vasculitidies can occur as idiopathic or secondary phenomena (e.g. complicating rheumatoid arthritis or systemic lupus erythematosis). In clinical practice, the most common vasculitis is **giant cell (temporal) arteritis**.

Large vessel vasculitis
Giant cell (temporal) arteritis

Giant cell arteritis (GCA) is a granulomatous inflammation of the aorta and large vessels, with a predilection for the extracranial branches of the carotid artery.

The most feared complication is of **visual disturbance**. Irreversible blindness occurs when the arteries supplying the retina or optic nerve head become involved (central retinal and posterior ciliary arteries); diplopia and ptosis may also occur. Visual loss may be the first symptom of GCA, but commonly it is preceded by temporal headache, scalp tenderness and jaw claudication.

In addition, 50% patients have a history of **polymyalgia rheumatica** (PMR) – an inflammatory disease causing classic shoulder and girdle muscular pain and stiffness, in the absence of weakness (which differentiates it from an inflammatory muscle disease).

The ESR (erythrocyte sedimentation rate) and CRP (C-reactive protein) are generally elevated, although disease in the presence of normal inflammatory markers has been reported. Temporal artery biopsy is notoriously unreliable due to the presence of skip lesions, but if positive is diagnostic.

Treatment

Treatment for both GCA and PMR is corticosteroid therapy. GCA requires high doses (30–80 mg prednisolone/day depending on the presence of visual symptoms), whereas PMR responds to much lower doses (e.g. 15 mg prednisolone/day). The clinical response is dramatic and steroids can be tapered according to the decline in symptoms and inflammatory markers. However, the majority of patients take 2 years or more to stop steroid therapy, so bone protection is mandatory and the use of azathioprine or methotrexate as steroid-sparing agents should be considered.

Takayasu arteritis

This rare vasculitis is commonest in women from the Far East, Central and South America and India. It is known as the 'pulseless disease' as large branches of the aorta become successively occluded. Symptoms are principally those of vascular ischaemia: claudication, visual disturbances and strokes, although many experience arthralgia. Bruits are common.

Diagnosis is by arteriography, and treatment requires corticosteroids and immunosuppression.

Medium vessel vasculitis
Polyarteritis nodosa

This necrotising vasculitis leads to aneurysm formation and predominantly involves vessels supplying the peripheral nerves, intestinal tract, kidney, skin and joints. Symptoms include marked constitutional upset, myalgias, orchitis and ischaemia (leading to vasculitic rashes, mononeuritis multiplex, renal failure, abdominal pain and coronary artery disease). It is associated with a marked inflammatory response and there is evidence of previous hepatitis B infection in up to 40% cases.

Diagnosis is by angiography, which reveals microaneurysms in the renal arterial tree and occlusions and irregular visceral arteries. Biopsy of affected tissue (e.g. skin or nerve) is occasionally undertaken. Treatment relies on corticosteroids and cytotoxics.

Kawasaki disease

This affects children, causing fever, conjunctival injection, fissuring/crusting of the lips, strawberry tongue, lymphadenopathy, erythema and desquamation of the hands. The vasculitis can affect all organs and the most feared complication is coronary arteritis.

Treatment is with aspirin and intravenous immunoglobulin.

Small vessel vasculitis

The small vessel vasculitidies are subdivided according to their association with ANCAs. The ANCA-positive vasculitidies are further subdivided according to staining patterns: cytoplasmic staining (cANCA) is directed against proteinase 3 and is associated with **Wegener's granulomatosis**. Perinuclear staining (pANCA) is directed against myeloperoxidase and is associated with **microscopic polyangiitis**.

ANCA-positive vasculitis
Wegener's granulomatosis

This is a systemic vasculitis with a classic triad of disease:
1 Upper airway (epistaxis, nasal crusting, outer and middle ear disease).
2 Lower airway (tracheobronchial stenosis, pulmonary haemorrhage).
3 Renal disease (glomerulonephritis, nephritic syndrome, renal failure).
Additional symptoms include marked constitutional upset, palpable purpura and livedo reticularis, arthralgia and mononeuritis multiplex.

Diagnosis relies on the clinical picture, raised inflammatory markers, positive cANCA (level fluctuates with disease activity), chest X-ray, CT chest ± biopsy and CT sinuses. Treatment is corticosteroid and cytotoxic therapy for the induction of remission and methotrexate or azathioprine for maintenance.

Microscopic polyangiitis

This predominantly causes a severe glomerulonephritis, but may lead to pulmonary haemorrhage, purpura, abdominal pain, arthralgias, peripheral neuropathy and cutaneous vasculitis. Investigations of choice are pANCA and renal biopsy, revealing a necrotising glomerulonephritis (the absence of granulomas differentiates this from Wegener's granulomatosis). Treatment is essentially as for Wegener's granulomatosis.

ANCA-negative vasculitis

The ANCA-negative vasculitidies include:
- **Hypersensitivity reactions**.
- **Henoch–Schönlein purpura**: purpura, arthritis, abdominal pain and IgA nephropathy.
- **Churg–Strauss syndrome**: asthma, peripheral eosinophilia, renal disease, gastrointestinal vasculitis and peripheral neuropathy (NB 25% of cases are cANCA positive).
- **Cryoglobulinaemia**: purpura, arthralgia and glomerulonephritis; associated with hepatitis C infection.
- Miscellaneous: infections and malignancy.

Tips

- Vasculitis is classified according to vessel size
- Small vessel vasculitis is divided into ANCA-positive (cANCA vs. pANCA) and ANCA-negative vasculitis

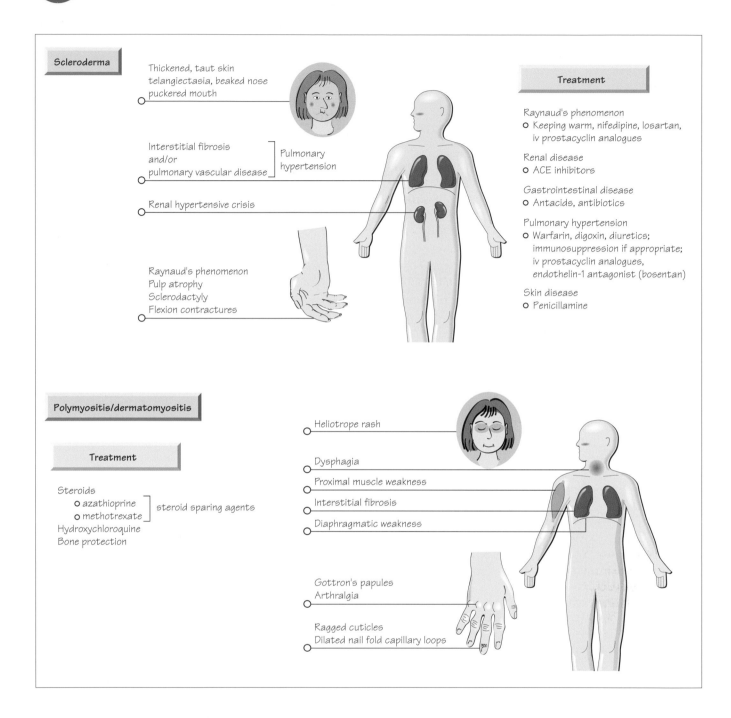

Scleroderma
- Thickened, taut skin telangiectasia, beaked nose puckered mouth
- Interstitial fibrosis and/or pulmonary vascular disease ⎤ Pulmonary hypertension
- Renal hypertensive crisis
- Raynaud's phenomenon
  Pulp atrophy
  Sclerodactyly
  Flexion contractures

Treatment

Raynaud's phenomenon
- Keeping warm, nifedipine, losartan, iv prostacyclin analogues

Renal disease
- ACE inhibitors

Gastrointestinal disease
- Antacids, antibiotics

Pulmonary hypertension
- Warfarin, digoxin, diuretics; immunosuppression if appropriate; iv prostacyclin analogues, endothelin-1 antagonist (bosentan)

Skin disease
- Penicillamine

Polymyositis/dermatomyositis
- Heliotrope rash
- Dysphagia
- Proximal muscle weakness
- Interstitial fibrosis
- Diaphragmatic weakness
- Gottron's papules
  Arthralgia
- Ragged cuticles
  Dilated nail fold capillary loops

Treatment

Steroids
- azathioprine ⎤ steroid sparing agents
- methotrexate
Hydroxychloroquine
Bone protection

Scleroderma

Scleroderma is a heterogeneous condition characterised by progressive fibrosis, widespread vascular disease and immunological abnormalities. It is divided into **limited cutaneous disease** (formerly known as CREST syndrome) and **diffuse cutaneous disease** (or systemic sclerosis).

Limited cutaneous disease

A relatively benign form of the disease affects the majority of patients with scleroderma syndromes. It is characterised by limited skin involvement (i.e. distance to knee and elbow) and a late appearance (if any) of visceral complications:

• **Cutaneous manifestations** are the result of overproduction of connective tissue, classically collagen. The skin becomes bound-down, taut, crease-free and hairless. The classic changes occur in the fingers (**sclerodactyly**) with a loss of finger pulp, the development of flexion contractures and reduced movement. Additional patterns of cutaneous disease include small, localised and circumscribed areas (morphoea), linear streaks frequently following a dermatomal distribution, or 'en coup de sabre', in which the face and scalp are involved. Calcinosis is also a common occurrence.

- **Vascular abnormalities** include Raynaud's phenomenon, telangiectasia and capillary nail fold abnormalities. Digital ischaemia and ulceration can occur late in the disease.
- **Gastrointestinal involvement** is limited to oesophageal dysmotility leading to dysphagia and reflux. More distal disease is rare.
- **Pulmonary hypertension** occurs as a result of interstitial fibrosis, pulmonary vascular disease or both.

Note that limited cutaneous scleroderma is now the preferred term for CREST syndrome (*c*alcinosis, *R*aynaud's phenomenon, *o*esophageal dysmotility, *s*clerodactyly and *t*elangiectasia).

Diffuse cutaneous disease

The complications of diffuse disease are universally more severe:
- **Cutaneous manifestations** spread proximally to include the trunk and face and patients develop a characteristic appearance with taut skin, a beaked nose and a tight mouth (microstomia) with restricted opening.
- **Vascular disease** is characterised by a renal obliterative endarteritis, which can precipitate a life-threatening renal hypertensive crisis.
- The entire **gastrointestinal tract** may become involved. The hypomobility generated by increasing fibrosis causes:
  reflux oesophagitis;
  small bowel malabsortion, including bacterial overgrowth;
  constipation and overflow diarrhoea due to colonic/rectal atony.
- In addition, the autoimmune condition primary biliary cirrhosis has an association with scleroderma and is a rare cause of diarrhoea.
- **Pulmonary hypertension** is also a feature of diffuse disease. As in the limited form, its onset is insidious, it is largely resistant to treatment and is a significant cause of mortality in this population.

Diagnosis and monitoring

The *diagnosis* of scleroderma relies on a thorough history and examination, with particular emphasis on the presence and severity of cutaneous and visceral involvement. Patients are antinuclear factor positive and disease-specific autoantibodies have been identified: diffuse/systemic disease is associated with antitopoisomerase-1 (Scl-70), limited disease with anti-centromere antibodies (ACA).

All patients should be *monitored* with regular outpatient assessment. Clinical evidence of end-organ damage should be sought and renal biochemistry and urinanalysis must be taken. Echocardiography and full lung function testing should be performed regularly as a screening tool for cardiopulmonary involvement.

Treatment

Scleroderma has no specific or curative treatment. Individual problems are tackled as follows:
- **Raynaud's phenomenon**: keeping warm and using vasodilators such as nifedipine and losartan.
- **Renal disease and hypertension**: ACE inhibition remains the treatment of choice. Dialysis may be necessary.
- **Gastrointestinal disease**: treatment of reflux disease is identical to normal treatment – antacids/alginates and proton-pump

inhibition. Antibiotics may assist in bacterial overgrowth and bulking agents can help with constipation.
- **Pulmonary hypertension**: all patients should receive warfarin, diuretics and digoxin. Interstitial disease may respond to immunosuppression with corticosteroids and cyclophosphamide.
- **Skin disease**: penicillamine and colchicine have been used to prevent the progression of cutaneous disease, and there are a number of trials assessing the efficacy of alkylating and immuno-modulating agents.

Polymyositis

Polymyositis is an inflammatory myopathy characterised by insidious muscle weakness and pain. Large proximal muscle groups are involved preferentially and patients have difficulty climbing stairs, rising from sitting or raising their arms above their heads. Shortness of breath may also occur as a result of diaphragmatic involvement, aspiration pneumonia or interstitial fibrosis.

Dermatomyositis refers to polymyositis in the presence of a characteristic rash that frequently precedes the myopathy. Papules develop over the metacarpophalangeal and proximal interphalangeal joints (Gottron's papules) with areas of linear erythema running the length of the finger's dorsal surface; the cuticles become ragged and dilated nail fold capillary loops become visible. Further cutaneous stigmata include a classically heliotrope rash across the eyelids and a macular eruption in a 'V' formation at the base of the neck and over the shoulders and back (the 'shawl' sign).

More unusual manifestations of disease include dysphagia, pericardial effusions and arthropathy.

Diagnosis

A firm diagnosis of polymyositis/dermatomyositis relies upon the history and examination, the presence of an inflammatory response and the triad of raised creatine kinase (CK) levels, abnormal electromyographs (EMG) and characteristic muscle biopsy. Many patients are antinuclear factor positive and the presence of the anti-Jo-1 autoantibody increases the likelihood of interstitial pulmonary fibrosis.

Treatment

Immunosuppression with high-dose corticosteroids forms the mainstay of treatment. The dose is gradually tapered according to clinical response and CK levels, and many patients will need up to 2 years of therapy. Up to a quarter of patients will require additional immunosuppression with azathioprine or methotrexate to obtain disease control. If the skin does not respond to steroid therapy, hydoxychloroquine may be added. Interstitial fibrosis is treated with steroids and cyclophosphamide.

Malignancy

Data suggest an increased incidence of malignancy in those with dermatomyositis (and polymyositis to a lesser degree). So a careful history and thorough clinical examination is mandatory. Chest X-ray, mammography and abdominal and pelvic ultrasounds would form the bare minimum of specialist investigations.

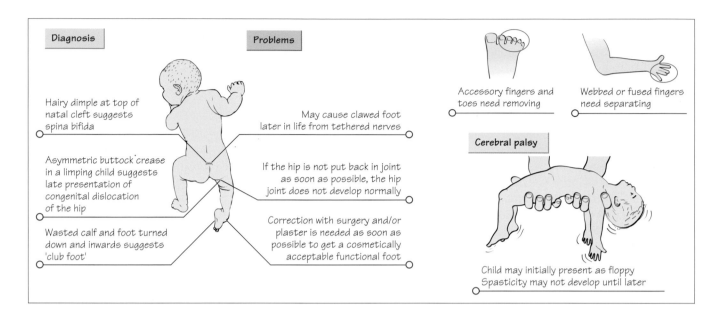

Antenatal and birth checks

Screening, genetic counselling, the withdrawal of teratogenic drugs and appropriate nutrition have greatly reduced the incidence of spina bifida and other congenital abnormalities in babies in the developed world. However, at birth all babies are checked for the most common abnormalities, which are unstable hips, club foot and abnormalities of the fingers and toes such as webbing, extra or absent digits.

Developmental dysplasia of the hip (DDH)

See Chapter 16.

Club foot (talipes equinovarus)

When the child is born, the foot is noted to be twisted down (equinus) and inwards (varus). This can either be a result of the position in the uterus (positional) or it can be congenital (failure of proper development of the calf and foot). If the problem is positional, then careful splinting will correct the problem. However, if the problem is anatomical (congenital), then surgical correction will be needed.

Webs, fusions and absent and accessory digits

Congenital abnormalities of the hand and foot can vary from slight webbing between two fingers or toes, through to complete absence of the limb. There may also be extra digits. Hands are very important in communication and not just for manipulation of tools, so cosmesis can be an important issue. Functionally in the hand, one of the most important needs is an opposable digit (a **thumb**). If this is absent then another digit may need to be rotated to take its place.

Artificial hands have proved very difficult to design because they require sensory feedback and exquisite control on grip pressure to come anywhere near the functionality of the normal hand.

Irritable hip

This is a common orthopaedic emergency because of the concern that serious pathology might be missed. The differentials are septic arthritis, Perthes' disease and slipped upper femoral epiphysis (see Chapter 16).

Knock-knees and bow legs

Children may be referred to the clinic with either knock-knees (**valgus**) or bow legs (**genu varus**). The degree of deformity is best measured by getting the child to stand with either their feet together (in the case of bow legs), or with their knees together (in the case of knock-knees). The distance between the medial condyles of the femur (in the case of bow legs) or the medial malleoli of the ankles (in the case of knock-knees) can then be measured. Most of these cases are benign and correct with time. All that is required is a regular check that the deformity is indeed improving as the child grows, combined with reassurance to the parents.

Fractures

Fractures heal rapidly in children; even if there is some malunion, the bones have great potential for remodelling, so angulation that would be quite unacceptable in an adult can be left in a child to heal itself. Children's bones are also quite flexible and may only break partially (a **greenstick fracture**). These tend to be stable

and only need protecting for a couple of weeks while they heal. However, there are two issues that need careful consideration:
1 The possibility of non-accidental injury.
2 The problem of fractures through epiphyseal growth plates.

Non-accidental injury

Certain fractures such as the spiral fracture of the femur in infants are highly suggestive of non-accidental injury, but there are many other features that may suggest that injuries have been caused deliberately:
• In the history there may be an inexplicable delay in presentation.
• The description of how the accident occurred does not fit with the nature of the injury (rolling off a sofa onto a carpet does not usually fracture the skull!).
• On examination the child is often quiet and watchful.
• There may be more bruises than expected, and they are sometimes of different ages suggesting multiple episodes of trauma.
• On X-ray there may be evidence of previous healed fractures, again suggesting that there has been more than one episode of trauma.

If there is any possibility of non-accidental injury, senior help should be sought.

Epiphyseal injuries

Fractures through the epiphyseal plate do not normally damage the blood supply (as the weakest zone is furthest away from the entry of the blood supply). However, if the fracture is displaced or enters the vascular zone the growth of the plate in that area may be arrested. If this is not recognised and corrected quickly the limb may end up deformed.

Cerebral palsy

The cause of cerebral palsy is not always known but can sometimes be a result of brain hypoxia secondary to birth trauma. Initially the child is floppy and then is slow to reach developmental landmarks. Spasticity then starts to develop, affecting variable amounts of the body. However severely affected the child, it is vital to remember that in many cases intelligence is unaffected, and no false assumptions should be made based on the problems the child has with taking in information or expressing themselves. Spasticity in muscles can cause abnormal bending of the spine and dislocation of joints, especially the hip.

Treatment is based on a careful blend of physiotherapy, orthotics and occasionally surgery to try to enable the child to get as much out of life as possible. This might involve fusion of the spine which enables them to sit straight up in a wheel chair, or a brace for a foot to enable them to walk better.

Tips

• If a child has one congenital abnormality, look for more
• Never assume that a child with cerebral palsy does not have normal intelligence
• Non-accidental injury has specific features in the history and examination
• Fractures in children are often partial and heal quickly
• Fractures through the growth plate may lead to growth arrest

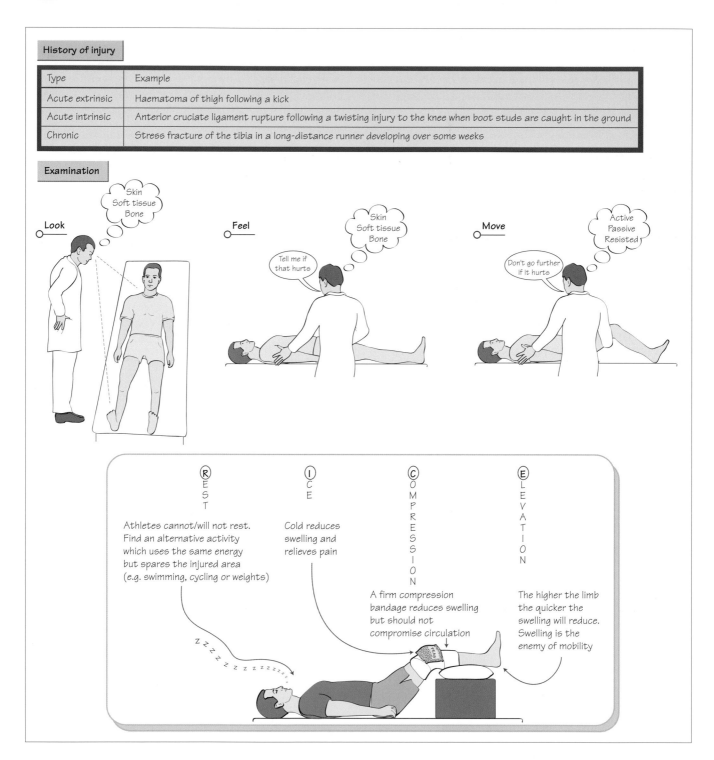

History of injury	
Type	Example
Acute extrinsic	Haematoma of thigh following a kick
Acute intrinsic	Anterior cruciate ligament rupture following a twisting injury to the knee when boot studs are caught in the ground
Chronic	Stress fracture of the tibia in a long-distance runner developing over some weeks

Definition

Sports medicine is at one end of the spectrum of musculo-skeletal disorders in that it relates to individuals who have very high expectations of their bodies, and who also have high motivation to get better as quickly as possible. Luckily, most of the patients are young so the potential for natural healing is also high.

History and examination

As usual, a good history can be very helpful. Careful listening to the athlete at the start of a consultation may reveal unexpected expectations. The injury may also be serving a purpose for changing training or as an honourable way out of sport altogether. It also allows classification of the injury into clear categories which simplify diagnosis.

Classification by presentation

In terms of diagnosis there are three types of presentation.

1 Acute extrinsic. The injury is caused by a direct blow and results in a bruise, a laceration or even a break.

2 Acute intrinsic. There is a sudden failure of a structure as a result of excessive load. This results in a tear of a muscle or ligament, a dislocation or a break in a bone.

3 Chronic. There is no single event that can be identified as the cause of the problem, more often there is a gradual onset. The problem may be inflammation of a tendon or its sheath or a stress fracture.

Sport specificity

Injuries tend to be associated with certain sports. The human body is not always well adapted to the loads applied. A few examples are given below.

Sport	Type of injury	Reason
Contact sports, e.g. football and rugby	Tear of the anterior cruciate ligament of the knee	Studded boots lock the foot to the ground imposing huge loads on the knee when the athlete turns or is tackled
Weight lifting	Spondylolisthesis of the spine	High repetitive loads to the base of the spine
Running	Stress fracture of the tibia	Repetitive high load from road running
Cricket	Shoulder, elbow and back problems	Repetitive loading especially when fast bowling
Ice hockey	Lacerations and teeth knocked out	High velocity impact. Sharp skates
Boxing	Acute and progressive brain damage	Multiple impacts to skull

Examination

This will often include watching the athlete performing their sport live. The purpose is to try to work out exactly what is happening to their body during performance of their sport. The examination will then follow the 'look, feel, move' system described in Chapters 3, 21.

Imaging

Dynamic imaging of the soft tissues is more likely to yield useful information than static imaging of the skeleton, so ultrasound may prove especially useful.

Treament
RICE (rest, ice, compression, elevation)

• *Rest* is not a meaningful concept for athletes. If one part of the body needs to be rested to allow healing to take place, then an equally strenuous programme of exercise which does not involve that part needs to be part of the prescription. Swimming and gym work can be very useful for runners with injured legs. Cycling can also be very good for unloading injured areas.

• *Ice* applied to injured areas (especially acute extrinsic injuries) appears to reduce inflammation and therefore speed recovery. Ice applied directly to the skin can cause a burn. Bags of frozen peas conform to the contours of a limb nicely.

• *Compression* used carefully can also reduce swelling and so speed recovery.

• *Elevation* speeds the recovery of swelling and inflammation.

Physiotherapy

This is the cornerstone of rapid and safe rehabilitation. Its role is to restore strength and mobility as fast as possible without allowing excessive exercise to cause further damage.

Injections

Injections of steroid into painful ligaments and joints can be used to try to reduce inflammation. The effect is usually short term and if more than two or three injections are given the steroid can weaken the tendon itself and cause a rupture. If local anaesthetic is used the injection can be used to try to diagnose the exact source of the pain or tenderness.

Fitness to return to sport

Athletes are fit to return to their sport when they are fit enough and confident enough to do so. For lower limb injuries the 'figure of eight' test is valuable (see p. 42).

Ligament tears

Partial tears can be allowed to heal without surgical intervention. Early movement with minimal loading stimulates healing while minimising pain and stiffness. Controlled exercises, hinged braces and removable splints may all have a role to play. Complete ligament tears may be best treated by surgical repair as this may speed up healing and return to full function.

Ruptured tendons

The blood supply to tendons is not good, so healing tends to be slow. However surgical repair is also not easy. This is especially true of the ruptured Achilles tendon which blights the career of so many middle-aged squash players.

Broken bones

Bones can be broken by direct trauma, or following repeated loading (stress fractures). Each **stress fracture** is associated with a certain sport. Running tends to produce fractures of the tibia (one cause of **shin splints**) or of the second metatarsal (the **'march' fracture**). Weight lifting can cause a fracture of the spine leading to a slip of the vertebral bodies on each other (**spondylolisthesis**). Stress fractures can be hard to see on X-ray and so may be difficult to diagnose. The gradual onset of symptoms can be confused with a simple strain or very rarely the onset of symptoms in a primary bone tumour.

Tips

• Classify sports injuries from the history
• RICE is useful for initial treatment
• The 'figure of eight' test is valuable for checking fitness
• Each sport is associated with specific injuries

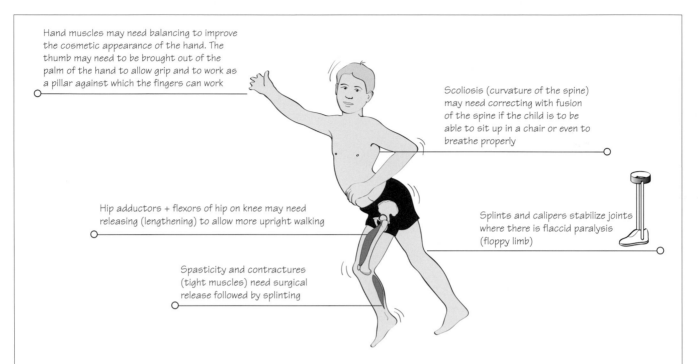

Hand muscles may need balancing to improve the cosmetic appearance of the hand. The thumb may need to be brought out of the palm of the hand to allow grip and to work as a pillar against which the fingers can work

Scoliosis (curvature of the spine) may need correcting with fusion of the spine if the child is to be able to sit up in a chair or even to breathe properly

Hip adductors + flexors of hip on knee may need releasing (lengthening) to allow more upright walking

Splints and calipers stabilize joints where there is flaccid paralysis (floppy limb)

Spasticity and contractures (tight muscles) need surgical release followed by splinting

Walking sticks

Help balance and increase confidence, especially out-of-doors, but rely on strong wrists. Aids may be needed for washing, shopping and house-work

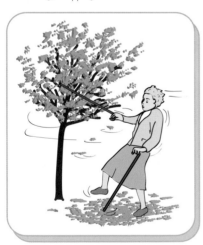

Crutches

Improve balance but also compensate for legs too weak to allow walking without extra help. Rely on strong elbows and shoulders. Aids will be needed and modifications to the house, e.g. stair lift, and a modified car may be needed

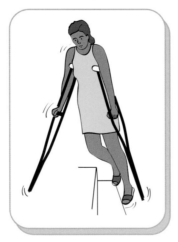

Wheel chair

Requires no strength in the lower limbs (except when transferring in and out of the chair). However, requires strength or stiffness in the spine to be able to sit up straight, and strength and co-ordination in the upper limbs if mobility is to be maintained without help or electric power and controls. Help may be needed around the house and modifications will be needed, ramps, etc.

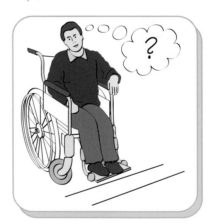

Neurological disorders

There are multitudes of neurological disorders that may present in an orthopaedic clinic. These can vary from polio, which has now almost disappeared from the developed world (but which once dominated orthopaedics), through to rare, familial disorders.

Classification

Neurological disorders can be divided into simple groups. There are those which are *static*, such as polio and cerebral palsy, and there are those which are *progressive*, such as Huntingdon's chorea. Secondly, there are those that affect only the *motor or sensory modality* (polio only affects motor nerves), or they can be *mixed motor and sensory*. The diagnosis and management is to a large degree based on this simple classification.

Management

The principles of management revolve around the same principles as in the rest of orthopaedics – the relief of pain, deformity and disability. In these cases disability is usually the main problem and physiotherapists, occupational therapists and social workers have a very major role to play in enabling these patients to live as full a life as possible.

Cerebral palsy

This is a non-progressive condition. The cause is unknown. It used to be thought that it was usually caused by birth trauma. More recently it appears that sometimes the damage may have already occurred *in utero*. The child is commonly a floppy baby with delayed 'milestones', and it is not for some time that the spasm develops that characterises cerebral palsy. These children are frequently of normal intelligence and great care must be taken not to assume that just because they are physically disabled and may have difficulty in communicating, that they are not of normal intelligence. The spasm of muscles reduces the ability of the child to produce powerful, coordinated movements, but also may produce fixed deformities of joints. These need to be avoided wherever possible.

Treatment goals in cerebral palsy

One of the key skills with a patient with a neurological disorder is to set realistic and useful goals. Devoting every waking hour for 5 years to getting a child to walk may be a triumph for everyone. But if this is achieved at a cost to their development in other ways, and if in a few years they go back off their feet, then this was not an appropriate goal. It might have been better devoting time and effort to developing good seating and training in the use of computers to help communication.

Orthotics and artificial limbs

This is the specialty of producing braces and splints designed to provide patients with support for limbs and artificial limbs. These can be temporary or permanent and may serve to reduce pain, improve function or even improve cosmesis. The traditional materials of leather and steel have been replaced with lightweight plastics, which conform so well in shape and colour that they can be almost invisible. They can be *static* (providing simple support) or *dynamic* (reproducing a movement that the patient is not capable of producing themselves).

When requesting imaging, you would be wise not to tell the radiographer what views you want, just explain the problem.

The same rules apply to an orthotist; it is their job to decide what splint is required. It is your job to explain the problem in terms of pain, deformity and disability, so that they can decide on the best way of managing the problem.

Dilemma of limb reconstruction versus early amputation

Severely injured limbs can pose a difficult clinical dilemma. Should a long reconstruction programme be started with an uncertain result, or would a better result be obtained by an early amputation with quick discharge from hospital and return back to normal life. As fast as new techniques are developed for reconstructing severely damaged limbs, new designs of prosthesis are appearing which are strong, cosmetically acceptable and give very good function, especially in the lower limb. Upper limb prostheses are hampered by the fact that no artificial limb can come near to the function of a normal limb that has feeling and which can use that feeling to control grip.

Sensory loss

However, if sensory function is unlikely to return because of permanent damage to sensory nerves, then **amputation** of a lower limb is strongly indicated. This is because if there is no protective sensation, then sores will develop which will ulcerate, and which may even lead to septicaemia. Amputation may also be the most appropriate route if there is no muscle power to stabilise joints, as this too severely reduces the functionality of a limb.

Modern methods of reconstruction

Bone transport using the **Ilizarov fixator** has now made it possible to grow bone across large defects in long bones. Similarly, **vascularised flaps** allow large soft tissue defects of muscle, as well as skin, to be covered. However, all these procedures are time-consuming and difficult to perform. If they fail the patient is left depressed and will have been in hospital for so long that their chances of return to normal life have effectively been destroyed. In retrospect an early amputation may have been the best option.

Modern orthotics

Below-knee prostheses are now light and strong. They are cosmetically almost indistinguishable from a normal leg and allow the patient to run, dance and take an active part in life. Above-knee amputations are more difficult as the knee hinge is more difficult to manage and the fit that can be obtained onto the thigh may be more difficult than the shin where there is less fat. Even so, a properly fashioned above-knee prosthesis can prove highly functional.

Tips

- Children with cerebral palsy start floppy then go spastic
- Goals need to be chosen appropriate to intelligence and mobility
- Artificial limbs are improving as fast as limb reconstruction techniques, so early amputation and rapid rehabilitation must remain a treatment option

Orthopaedics in the elderly

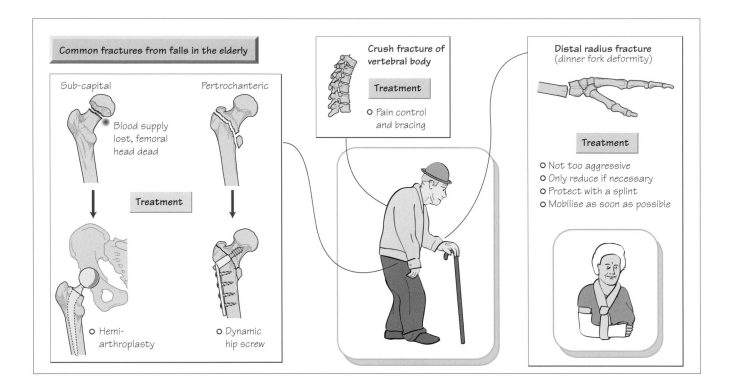

Introduction

The population of the developed world is aging rapidly. The problems of the elderly have come to dominate orthopaedic and trauma services. There are a number of special problems:

- Falls, both because of weakness and loss of balance.
- Fractures, because of falls and because bones are weakened by osteoporosis.
- Osteoarthritis.
- Malignant disease, producing pathological fractures.
- Foot problems, causing painful bunions and corns.
- The rotator cuff around the shoulder weakens and may tear.
- Arthritis in the spine may cause symptoms of nerve root compression.

Old people value their independence just like everyone else but rehabilitation after an accident becomes increasingly difficult with age. Accidents need to be prevented if possible, and treated quickly and efficiently when they do, otherwise even a trivial injury can become the 'straw which breaks the camel's back' precipitating an independent patient into one who is in permanent care.

Fractures caused by osteoporosis

Bone density falls with age, especially in thin women after the menopause. Trivial falls can then lead to major fractures. The commonest sites of these osteoporotic fractures are the wrist, spine and neck of the femur.

Wrist

At the wrist the fracture involves impaction (crushing) and bending backwards of the forearm bones just above the wrist joint, sometimes called the 'dinner fork' deformity or **Colles' fracture**. The fracture tends to be stable because of the impaction and some surgeons feel that it is best not to reduce the fracture (and so make it unstable), but let it heal quickly in its new position. This offers the best chance of preserving the patient's independence as they may only need a simple splint for comfort for a couple of weeks if the fracture is left alone, rather than a full plaster for over a month if it is reduced.

Spine

Crush fractures of the spine are stable and rarely compress nerves, although they can be very painful. Treatment is symptomatic.

Neck of the femur

Fractures of the neck of the femur are very different. There are two types:

1 The high neck fracture interrupts the blood supply to the head, so if it is displaced the head dies and needs to be replaced with a **hemi-arthroplasty** (half a hip joint).

2 If the fracture is low in the neck then the blood supply to the head will remain intact but the fracture will need treating with internal fixation. The device used (a **dynamic hip screw**) holds the fracture while allowing the margins to compress together. This holds the fracture steady and stimulates rapid healing.

The great advantage of these two techniques is that they allow the patient to get up and start walking at once, so minimising the chance of the patient losing their independence or developing some other illness associated with prolonged bed rest.

Osteoarthritis

The cause of osteoarthritis is not known but once the articular cartilage is damaged, the deterioration can be rapid. The joint becomes stiff and painful and may be fixed in a position that is not ideal for function. For example, both the hip and the knee tend to become fixed in flexion making it difficult for the patient to walk upright.

Joint replacement should primarily reduce the pain but can also improve range of movement, converting someone who is house-bound, dependent on others and in pain to an outgoing, independent, cheerful person once again. The joints now last for around 10–15 years and can then be changed (revised) to prolong a good quality of life even further.

Metastases

Primary tumours of bone are rare but many tumours can metastasise to bone. If the lesions can be spotted early, radiotherapy can be used to prevent further bone destruction. If the bone is so eroded that it is at imminent risk of breaking, or has in fact already broken, fixation with a locked **intramedullary nail** will reduce the pain and prevent the patient from being confined to bed during the whole of their terminal illness.

Bunions, corns and metatarsalgia

The feet become less and less able to cope with pressure and rubbing as patients get older. Deformities that were once correctable may also become fixed producing even more problems from shoes. The treatment of choice is usually non-surgical by providing insoles and special shoes which reduce excessive pressure. Surgery to correct deformity needs to be embarked on with great care as healing may be slow.

Rotator cuff

Extra bone forming on the outer edge of the acromion may rub on the rotator cuff producing pain as the inflamed area passes in under this sharp shelf of bone. If the rotator cuff is overloaded or subject to repeated rubbing from impingement it may tear, making it difficult or even impossible for the patient to lift their arm above their head because the **supraspinatus tendon** has snapped. Impingement can be treated by trimming the beak of bone, but tears of the rotator cuff are difficult to repair in the elderly because of the poor blood supply.

Spinal stenosis

Narrowing of the spinal canal or of the gaps between the facet joint and the disc where the spinal nerve leaves the canal, present with back pain and spinal stenosis. This commonly presents as pain on walking for some distance, especially downhill when the extension of the spine narrows the canal even further. Surgical treatment to open up the narrowed areas is difficult and may not always be successful.

Tips

- Elderly patients need and deserve early treatment of their common orthopaedic problems to preserve independent existence
- Healing, especially in the feet, is slow
- There are two types of fractured neck of the femur with completely different treatments
- Tumours in bones are metastases

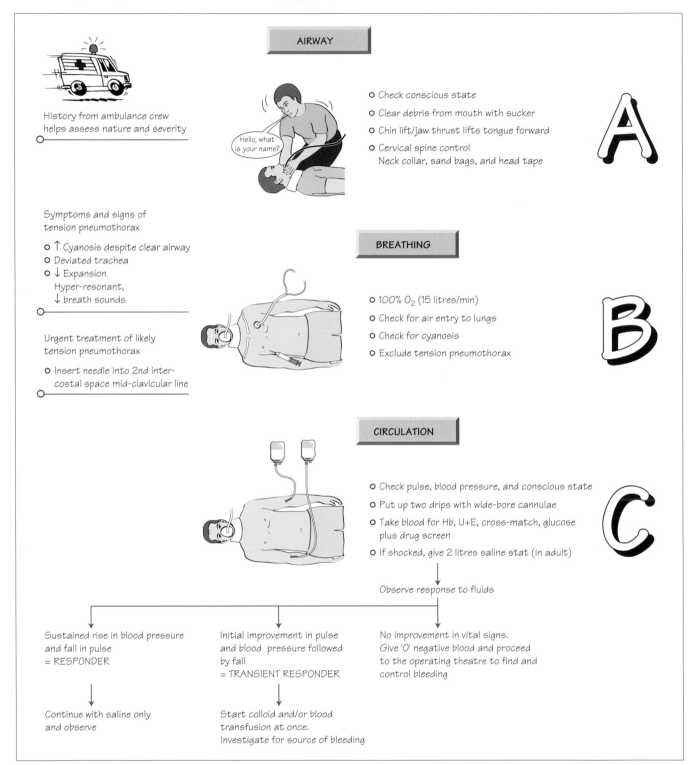

AIRWAY

- Check conscious state
- Clear debris from mouth with sucker
- Chin lift/jaw thrust lifts tongue forward
- Cervical spine control
  Neck collar, sand bags, and head tape

History from ambulance crew helps assess nature and severity

Hello, what is your name?

Symptoms and signs of tension pneumothorax

- ↑ Cyanosis despite clear airway
- Deviated trachea
- ↓ Expansion
  Hyper-resonant,
  ↓ breath sounds

Urgent treatment of likely tension pneumothorax

- Insert needle into 2nd inter-costal space mid-clavicular line

BREATHING

- 100% O_2 (15 litres/min)
- Check for air entry to lungs
- Check for cyanosis
- Exclude tension pneumothorax

CIRCULATION

- Check pulse, blood pressure, and conscious state
- Put up two drips with wide-bore cannulae
- Take blood for Hb, U+E, cross-match, glucose plus drug screen
- If shocked, give 2 litres saline stat (in adult)

Observe response to fluids

Sustained rise in blood pressure and fall in pulse
= RESPONDER

Initial improvement in pulse and blood pressure followed by fall
= TRANSIENT RESPONDER

No improvement in vital signs. Give 'O' negative blood and proceed to the operating theatre to find and control bleeding

Continue with saline only and observe

Start colloid and/or blood transfusion at once. Investigate for source of bleeding

Introduction

Patients involved in serious accidents are becoming rarer and rarer in developed countries, but are more likely than ever to arrive at hospital alive however severe their injuries. This is a result of better communications and improved pre-hospital care. Serious accidents often involve young people with great potential for healing and a long productive life ahead of them. The stakes are high and the first few hours have a profound effect on the long-term outcome. Working to a system allows a team to work quickly and efficiently. This chapter presents a simple system for this initial management.

History

The patient may not be able to give a history, but a description from the paramedics of the energy involved in the accident will give a clue to the likely type and severity of the patient's injuries.

As a general rule if there is one significant injury then there are likely to be more, so always do a complete survey in a seriously injured patient.

Initial management

The initial approach to a seriously injured patient is given by the acronym **ABC** followed by **D** and **E**.

Airway and neck stabilisation (A)

• Start by asking the patient for their name. If they can answer then you have confirmed that their **airway** (A), **breathing** (B) and **conscious** state are all reasonable.
• While this is being done someone should be taking control of the neck with 'in-line immobilisation', prior to the neck being stabilised with a stiff collar, sandbags and tape, just in case there is an unstable fracture of the cervical spine.
• If the patient does not answer, start by checking the mouth and throat for obstructions, broken teeth and other material. A sucker is safer than a finger, as a semiconscious patient may bite.
• A chin lift or jaw thrust will lift the tongue forward from out of the throat if this is the cause of the obstruction.

Breathing (B)

Start giving 100% oxygen at 15 l/min (full bore). Check for breathing and air entry into the lungs by looking for chest movement and listening to the lungs. If the patient does not appear to be breathing start bagging them with an Ambu bag and prepare for intubation. If the patient's colour is not good, check again that the airway is clear, then check for a **tension pneumothorax**. The most obvious sign will be a deviated trachea.

If a tension pneumothorax is suspected then a blue needle needs to be introduced into the second intercostal space in the mid-clavicular line. If the diagnosis is correct the patient's condition should improve at once, and a chest drain can then be inserted later. If not little has been lost.

Circulation (C)

Two wide-bore cannulae should be introduced, one into each antecubital vein (front of the elbow). Bloods are drawn for cross-match, full blood count, electrolytes, glucose and drug screen. Two litres of Hartmann's solution can then be given as quickly as they can be transfused (stat) if the patient is in deep shock. This fluid challenge will give a clue to the seriousness of the situation and allow you to plan the next stage. If the patient's blood pressure rises and their pulse falls back to normal levels and then they remain stable, the patient is a 'responder'. No further aggressive action needs to be taken for the moment, although blood should still be cross-matched.

If the patient improves but then starts to deteriorate again, then a plasma expander is needed urgently and further investigations are necessary to find the source of the bleeding. 'O'-negative or type-specific blood may be ordered to save time on the cross-match. Up to 8 units should be ordered in the first instance.

If there is no response to the fluid challenge then the patient needs 'O'-negative blood at once and surgery to try to stem the haemorrhage at once. The main sites for heavy bleeding are the chest, abdomen and pelvis.

Disability

Check and record the patient's conscious state using the Glasgow coma scale (see Chapter 39). At every stage keep rechecking the ABC, especially if the patient's condition starts to deteriorate.

Exposure

Remove all clothes and check the patient from top to toe using the 'look, feel, move' system (see Chapters 3, 21). Log-roll the patient to check the back as well, looking all over the body for cuts, bruises and deformity. A rectal and vaginal examination will also be needed, to check for pelvic injuries. A urinary catheter can then be safely inserted and used to monitor the patient's perfusion.

Repetition

Every check must be repeated again and again. Patients can 'go off' at any time and if they do it is commonly something simple like their airway, breathing or circulation that is causing the problem and which needs correcting.

Investigations like CT scans should only be undertaken once the patient's condition is stable so a further check of ABC will be needed before the patient is moved.

Recording

All findings should be clearly recorded with the time when they were observed. It is often a gradual change in an observation which tells you more about what is happening to a patient than a single value.

Check

Before the patient leaves the resuscitation room, every injury however small must have been found, measured and noted, and an appropriate care plan written. Once the patient has been transferred to the ward, it is all too easy for injuries to be missed and what might have been a trivial injury at the start (e.g. a dislocated finger) now may become a major impediment to return to normal existence.

Tips

• Rescue workers can give a good estimate of the energy involved in an accident
• Use ABC
• A sucker is better than a finger for clearing the mouth
• If there is one significant injury then look for more
• Working to a system allows the whole team to work quickly and efficiently
• Record all your findings clearly, looking for trends
• Keep going back to check ABC

Wound management

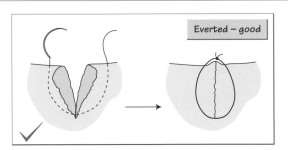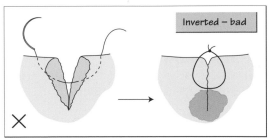

If you cannot completely clean a dirty wound, pack it and leave it open

Everted – good

Inverted – bad

Your stitch should reach to the floor of the wound and take more tissue deep than superficially
Then, when the stitch is tightened, the wound will evert and there will be no dead space

General assessment

Carry out a rapid general assessment of the whole patient to make sure that their airway, breathing and circulation are satisfactory (ABC, then D and E; see Chapter 34) before focusing in on the presenting injury.

History

Try to find out how long ago the wound occurred and whether the object that caused it was likely to be clean or contaminated, or even whether any noxious chemicals or electrical burn may be involved (see Chapter 37). Clean cuts that occurred recently are managed completely differently from dirty wounds or those that may already be infected.

Examination

Check distal neurovascular status. The sooner that damage to a vessel or nerve can be identified, the better the chance that a repair can be performed and the function of the limb saved.

Investigation

An X-ray is useful to exclude fracture or dislocation. Two views need to be taken at right angles to each other, centred on the injured area. The entry wound can be marked with a paper clip taped to the skin.

Cleaning

Wounds must not be closed if there is any chance that they might become infected. Copious volumes of saline should be used to wash the wound out – dead and contaminated tissue must be removed.

If at the end of your best efforts you cannot be sure that the wound is clean then pack it and review the situation daily until you are sure it is clean. Then, and only then, should you close it.

Exploration

Good light is needed to inspect a wound properly. Local or general anaesthesia may also be needed, so wounds are best explored in an operating theatre. If the limb was in a different position when the injury occurred to its position when the examination is performed, it is easy to miss the depth of the wound. For example, it is also easy to miss that the knuckle joint has been penetrated in an injury from a punch onto the teeth of an opponent. If the hand is examined with the fingers extended, the skin wound appears to be well away from the knuckle itself.

Repair

Damaged nerves, vessels, ligaments and bones should be repaired as soon as possible, but the first priority must be to remove non-viable tissue and then to ensure that there is adequate skin and soft tissue cover to ensure infection-free healing.

Tetanus

Prophylaxis against tetanus must be up to date or tetanus toxoid will be needed. Prophylactic antibiotics may also be given but are no substitute for proper wound cleaning.

Pain relief and rehabilitation

Wounds are painful and can lead to wasting and stiffness if no effort is made to ensure that the patient builds up muscle strength and mobility as quickly as possible. This is especially important in the hand where the role of the physiotherapist is crucial.

Stitching

When stitching a wound make sure the edges are everted.

Tips

- Check ABC and for other wounds
- Test distal neurovascular status
- Ultrasound may be better than an X-ray for finding glass
- Do not close a wound unless you are sure it is clean
- Exploration of a wound is best done in an operating theatre
- Protection against tetanus needs to be checked

Superficial skin loss

Superficial skin loss will heal well provided there is no dirt left in it and it does not become infected. The donor site of a split skin graft heals in a similar way

Skin defect from congenital abnormalities

Tissue expanders can slowly stretch the skin to create spare skin for reconstruction

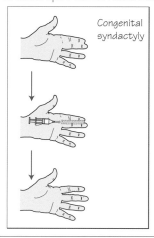

Congenital syndactyly

Full thickness skin loss

If the wound cannot be closed and there is healthy soft tissues in the floor of the wound, a split skin graft can be harvested elsewhere on the body and used to provide cover. The scar does not look good and cannot tolerate heavy use, e.g. sole of the foot

Large areas of full thickness loss

Split skin grafts can be 'meshed' to increase the area which each piece can cover. Skin cells can be grown in culture to cover very large areas

Exposed bone

A vascular graft of skin and muscle is needed. Sometimes it is possible to rotate a flap locally, covering the donor area with a split skin graft. Otherwise a vascularised free graft will need to be taken from elsewhere on the body (usually the back) and connected into the local blood supply using micro-surgery. The donor site is closed or grafted

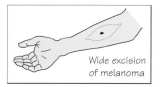

Wide excision of melanoma

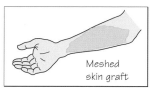

Meshed skin graft

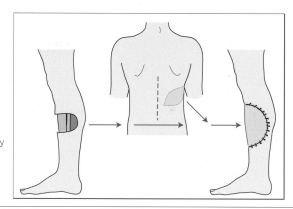

Plastic surgery is the craft of moving skin and soft tissues to repair damage or to improve appearance and function.

The skin provides a crucial function preventing excess fluid from leaving the body and infection from entering the body. Soft tissues are also necessary to provide a substrate for healthy skin. When skin and soft tissues are lost due to trauma or because diseased tissue has been excised, it may not be possible to simply close the defect. Exposed bone and ligaments will become infected if they are not covered, while soft tissues left to heal of their own accord may leave ugly scars which hamper normal function when they contract as part of the healing process.

• **Superficial defects (grazes and partial thickness burns).** In these cases the skin heals from nests of **epithelial cells** growing out from hair follicles where they were protected from the original trauma. Healing is reasonable providing the damaged area is cleaned and kept free of infection.

• **Full thickness defects (complete loss of skin with intact soft tissues beneath).** Surgeons use the skin's ability to heal partial thickness defects to harvest epithelial skin which can then be used as a **split skin graft** to cover a full thickness defect. The graft can be meshed to cover a larger area and will stimulate rapid healing without contracture, although the scar is not attractive and the resistance of the graft area to abrasion is poor. For very large defects it is now possible to culture epithelial cells from the patient and use these to 'seed' the growth of an epithelial cover.

• **Complete soft tissue loss (exposed bone).** Skin and underlying vascularised muscle will be needed to cover these defects. If it is possible to rotate nearby skin and muscle to cover the defect while maintaining its blood supply, then this pedicle graft will be the best option. Normally it is possible to dissect out an area of skin and underlying muscle from a part of the body where it can be spared. This **vascularised graft** is then plumbed into its new site, using microsurgery to connect its arterial supply and venous drainage to the local blood supply.

Tips

• Decide depth of defect and plan treatment accordingly
• The body needs skin cover to prevent fluid loss and infection
• If infection is allowed to set in, the wound effectively becomes deeper
• Don't close dirty wounds

---

37 Burns

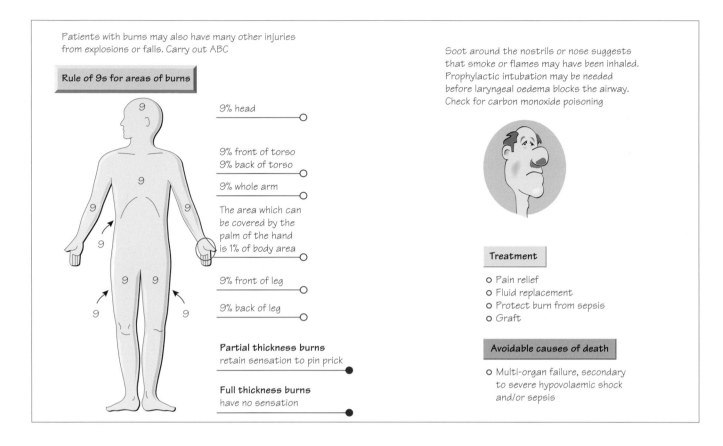

Patients with burns may also have many other injuries from explosions or falls. Carry out ABC

Rule of 9s for areas of burns

9% head

9% front of torso
9% back of torso

9% whole arm

The area which can be covered by the palm of the hand is 1% of body area

9% front of leg

9% back of leg

Partial thickness burns
retain sensation to pin prick

Full thickness burns
have no sensation

Soot around the nostrils or nose suggests that smoke or flames may have been inhaled. Prophylactic intubation may be needed before laryngeal oedema blocks the airway. Check for carbon monoxide poisoning

Treatment

○ Pain relief
○ Fluid replacement
○ Protect burn from sepsis
○ Graft

Avoidable causes of death

○ Multi-organ failure, secondary to severe hypovolaemic shock and/or sepsis

History

If the patient cannot tell you what happened, then the paramedics should be able to advise on whether the burn was caused by heat, chemicals, electric shock or a combination of all of these. They will also be able to warn if other trauma is involved (such as a jump from a burning building).

Airway and breathing

• If smoke was involved or if there is any sign of soot or burns around the mouth or nose, then damage to the airway from **smoke inhalation** must be considered.

• Smoke may contain carbon monoxide.

• Toxic fumes in the smoke may also have caused chemical damage to the lungs. This may lead to a rapid onset of **pulmonary oedema** with a fall in blood gases and the need for assisted ventilation.

• If the patient has actually breathed in flames, damage to the lining of the upper airway will lead to swelling of the glottis. **Stridor** will be the first sign – followed rapidly by **complete airway obstruction**. It is safest to perform endotracheal intubation early, as it can be almost impossible to find the vocal cords once oedema has set in. Otherwise, an emergency tracheostomy will be needed.

Circulation

Patients with burns lose large volumes of fluid by exudation and evaporation. These fluids need to be replaced if circulation is to be maintained and renal failure avoided. A cut-down may be needed to obtain good venous access, for crystalloids, colloids and even blood transfusion. In severe cases a urinary catheter and a central venous line will be needed to monitor the state of the circulation so that the appropriate volume of fluids can be given.

Protection and pain relief

Exposed wounds lose fluid, cool the patient by evaporation, are very painful and are at risk of becoming infected. Any foreign material embedded in the wound will need removing, but at this stage it is only important to make sure that noxious chemicals are washed away and any smouldering material is cooled down so that the burn does not extend. The burns are best covered with cling-film or some other non-stick conforming dressing covering some kind of antiseptic cream such as silver sulfazine.

Electrical burns

High voltage electric shocks will traverse the patient's body leaving only a small entry and exit burn visible externally, even when there is extensive internal damage. An electrocardiograph (ECG) will be needed to exclude myocardial damage; compartment syndrome is also a risk in the limbs.

Assessing the severity of the burn

The severity of burns is determined by the area involved and the depth of the burns.

Area

In the first instance, the area of the body surface that is burnt is estimated using two techniques:

1 The area covered by the hand of the patient is estimated to be 1% of the total body surface area.

2 The **rule of 9s** is more useful in extensive burns. Nine areas of the body each make up approximately 9% of the total surface area.

Depth

Superficial burns

- Superficial burns cause reddening or blistering of the skin.
- Sensation is preserved and the prognosis for recovery is good provided sepsis does not set in.
- The deepest parts of the dermis – around the pores and hair follicles – are preserved and act as a source of cells from which the rest of the epithelium regenerates.
- Fluid loss can be considerable but once healing has occurred scarring is minimal.

Full thickness burns

- Full thickness burns completely destroy the dermis and the tissues beneath.
- They can be distinguished from superficial burns because there is no sensation when the area is tested by pinprick.
- The dead tissue must be removed as it is a focus for infection. Dead tissue is shaved off layer by layer until fresh bleeding is obtained.

- Then a decision needs to be made as to how the area is to be covered. Meshed **split skin grafts** provide a good source of cover, especially for large areas in the first instance. However they tend to give a poor result cosmetically.
- Once the patient has recovered from the initial trauma it may be decided to replace the initial grafts with **full thickness grafts** or even free flaps, especially in areas where appearances are important (e.g. the face), or where heavy wear is likely to ulcerate a split skin graft (e.g. palm of the hand).
- Full thickness burns left to heal of their own accord shrink down as they heal, producing contractures that can destroy function and look very ugly.

Sepsis

Sepsis in a superficial burn can convert it to a full thickness lesion, while sepsis in a graft can lead to death of the graft. If the sepsis then spreads, septicaemia may lead to **multiorgan failure**, the commonest cause of death after burns if the patient survives the first few hours. Full sterile precautions, proper surgical cleaning and prophylactic antibiotics all play a role in trying to prevent infection.

Fluid balance

Burn patients lose large volumes of fluid and go into renal failure if these fluids are not replaced. Colloid and blood, not just crystalloid, may be needed to maintain the extracellular fluid compartment volume, and prevent shutdown of the kidneys.

Mortality

The chance of a patient surviving a burn decreases with the increasing area and depth of the burn and the age of the patient.

Tips

- Smoke inhalation may need urgent intubation
- Burns patients need to be kept well hydrated
- Sepsis needs to be avoided if at all possible

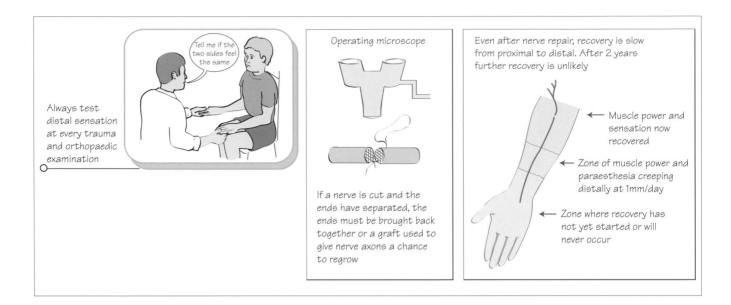

Always test distal sensation at every trauma and orthopaedic examination

Tell me if the two sides feel the same

Operating microscope

If a nerve is cut and the ends have separated, the ends must be brought back together or a graft used to give nerve axons a chance to regrow

Even after nerve repair, recovery is slow from proximal to distal. After 2 years further recovery is unlikely

Muscle power and sensation now recovered

Zone of muscle power and paraesthesia creeping distally at 1mm/day

Zone where recovery has not yet started or will never occur

Diagnosis

Nerve injuries are easily missed in the turmoil of major injuries, or if the patient is drunk or upset. Testing should be done by comparing sides, not by asking the patient to close their eyes and then asking if they can feel you touching them. The second method is notoriously unreliable, while the first reliably warns you when a full formal neurological examination may be needed.

As a general rule penetrating wounds in the hand have always damaged a nerve until otherwise proven. Similarly, in the neck and spine it is best to assume the worst (there is an unstable fracture with potential for further nerve damage) until this possibility has been actively excluded (see Chapter 34). Some nerves, like the lateral popliteal (foot drop) and the radial nerve (wrist drop), are especially susceptible to injury because of their position.

Peripheral nerve injuries
Minor injuries

Minor compression of a peripheral nerve can lead to loss of function of that nerve for some days or even weeks. The nerve fibres are intact and physiological function returns in time without any need for tissue healing.

Severe injuries

• **Incomplete severing of the nerve**. In more severe injuries some of the fibres (axons) in the nerve may be severed but the overall structure of the nerve may remain intact. In these cases the axon proximal and distal to the cut dies (Wallerian degeneration), leaving the tunnel of Schwann cells (if it was a myelinated fibre) through which the fibre originally passed. This tunnel acts as a guide for a new nerve fibre to grow back at around 1 mm/day. The progress of the regrowth can sometimes

be traced by tapping your finger over the path of the healing nerve. When you tap over the tip of the new growing fibre, the patient will experience electric shocks running down the arm.

• **Complete severing of the nerve**. An injury that completely separates the ends of the nerve cannot heal unless those nerve ends are brought back into close contact, preferably with the nerve fibre ends correctly aligned with each other. Otherwise there is a danger that the regenerating axon tip will set off down the wrong track thus compromising the function of the nerve. The repair of the nerve is best performed under an operating microscope to obtain accurate opposition; if there is a segment of nerve missing, then a nerve graft may be created from a length of another less important nerve to act as a guide to the regenerating nerve fibres.

Nerve recovery

• Nerve recovery tends not to be so good in the elderly, where the nerve fibres are very long, and where the nerve has a mixture of sensory and motor fibres.

• While waiting for nerves to regrow there is important work to be done by physiotherapists in preventing muscles from wasting, and joints from stiffening up.

• If there is also sensory loss then these areas may need to be protected from unnoticed damage, especially burns, which may lead to ulceration.

• Recovery of sensation can be tested using hair bristles of differing stiffness (noting the softest that the patient can feel), and by testing **two point discrimination** (the smallest distance between two pricks that can be distinguished as separate points).

Injuries to the central nervous system

The peripheral nervous system extends out from the spinal ganglia (dorsal for sensory, ventral for motor). The rest of the nervous system (pre-ganglionic) consists of the brain and the spinal cord. Injury to these nerves leads initially to a state of **spinal shock** (concussion) when the nerves fail to work at all. The spinal shock wears off over a period of hours or days and it is only then that the true extent of the damage to the nervous system will become apparent.

In spinal cord injuries, the finding that there is sparing of the central sacral roots is the first indication that there may be some recovery of function and that the transection of the cord is not complete. The central nervous system has very little capacity for tissue healing but has an extraordinary ability to reorganise so that damaged tissue is by-passed. This process takes time and this plasticity decreases with age.

As the spinal shock wears off patients may get a false hope of recovery from the fact that their muscles are starting to contract. However, this may be **spasticity** setting in, a result of complete and irreversible nerve damage.

Brachial plexus injuries

If the arm is dragged down by a high energy impact (such as a fall from a high speed motorcycle), there may a tearing injury to the nerves coming from the neck through the brachial plexus into the arm. The injury can be a mixture of:
• Pre-ganglionic damage where the nerve roots actually pull out the ganglia.
• Post-ganglionic damage where the brachial plexus is torn apart.

Repair is likely to be at best a limited success, and is technically very difficult. The patient is unfortunately often left with severe and intractable pain in a useless arm. The pain is very difficult to treat and is not helped by amputation. The patient may become suicidal as a result.

Rehabilitation
• Long periods of rehabilitation will be needed if a patient who has suffered a significant injury to the brain or spinal cord is to have the best chance of returning to a full independent life.
• Head injuries can result in significant behaviour changes, memory loss and problems with concentration, as well as problems with spasticity.
• Permanent sensory loss means that the patient must learn to move regularly if bedsores are to be avoided, as once these have started they can be very difficult to treat.

Tips

• If the tendon is damaged in a finger injury then the digital nerves are also probably injured
• Nerve ends need bringing together (if necessary with a graft) if any nerve recovery is to occur
• After 2 years there is unlikely to be further nerve recovery
• Stiffness and wasting need to be minimised while waiting for nerve recovery

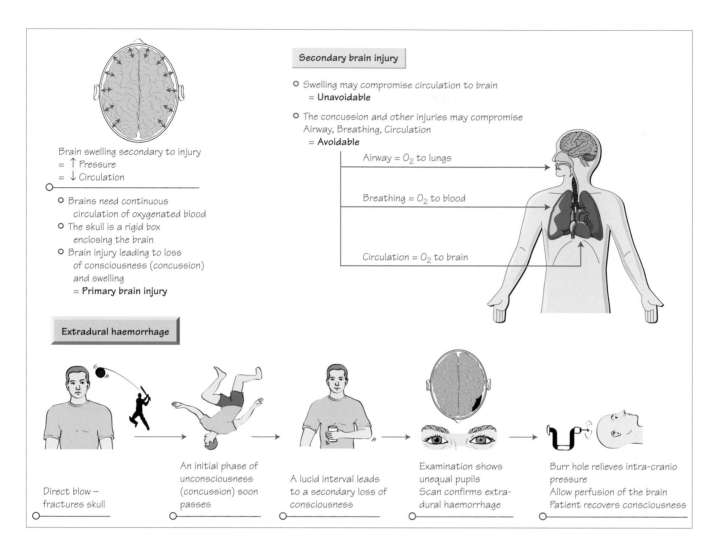

Brain swelling secondary to injury
= ↑ Pressure
= ↓ Circulation

○ Brains need continuous
   circulation of oxygenated blood
○ The skull is a rigid box
   enclosing the brain
○ Brain injury leading to loss
   of consciousness (concussion)
   and swelling
   = **Primary brain injury**

Secondary brain injury

○ Swelling may compromise circulation to brain
   = **Unavoidable**

○ The concussion and other injuries may compromise
   Airway, Breathing, Circulation
   = **Avoidable**

Airway = O_2 to lungs

Breathing = O_2 to blood

Circulation = O_2 to brain

Extradural haemorrhage

Direct blow –
fractures skull

An initial phase of
unconsciousness
(concussion) soon
passes

A lucid interval leads
to a secondary loss of
consciousness

Examination shows
unequal pupils
Scan confirms extra-
dural haemorrhage

Burr hole relieves intra-cranio
pressure
Allow perfusion of the brain
Patient recovers consciousness

Introduction

The brain is arguably the human's most precious organ. It is well protected by the skull, but it is large and heavy and so is prone to injury, especially from blows that rapidly accelerate and then decelerate it within the confines of the skull. Significant injuries to the brain lead to a temporary shut-down of higher functions (**concussion**). However, it must never be forgotten that unconsciousness can also be coma, or a result of stroke, hypoglycaemia, epilepsy or drugs. So, the loss of consciousness may have been the cause of the accident not the result.

The key to the management of most head injuries is ensuring that the brain remains well perfused in the post-injury and recovery period. Failure to keep the airway clear, the blood well oxygenated and the brain well perfused may lead to so-called 'secondary injury' to the brain. This damage should be avoidable.

Initial management

As in any serious injury the initial management is **ABC** (see Chapter 34) followed by an assessment of conscious state and a check for any other injuries. Patients with serious head injuries may not be making any effort to breathe or may have lost their gag reflex. Early endotracheal intubation may be needed to keep the patient well oxygenated, and to protect the airway from inhalation.

Assessment of conscious state is made using the **Glasgow coma score** which gives marks for the best response in a set of different areas (response to verbal command, response to pain, eye movements). An early measure of the conscious state is valuable because it is any subsequent *change* in the conscious state, rather than the absolute level that guides further investigation and treatment. If the conscious state starts to deteriorate always check ABC before looking for neurological causes.

A scan of the brain is needed if intracranial bleeding is suspected but the patient must first be made safe to enter the scanner.

Types of head injury
Cuts on the scalp

These bleed profusely and can cause **hypovolaemic shock**. They should always be explored in case they lie over a fracture or even a penetrating wound into the brain itself.

Fractured skull

A fractured skull is of no great significance in itself unless it is depressed and fragments are pressing into the brain. However, it is an indication of the severity of trauma, and if close to a blood vessel may provoke an intracranial bleed. If the fracture is open then blood mixed with cerebrospinal fluid will flow out of the ear, nose or wound and prophylactic antibiotics need to be given to protect against meningitis.

Extradural haemorrhage

Fractures near cranial arteries – especially the middle meningeal artery (running up the side of the skull by the temple) – may tear the artery itself. This produces bleeding between the skull and the dural membrane, which will slowly start to compress the brain over a period of hours. Classically the patient has a short period of unconsciousness (concussion) followed by a recovery of faculties. However, some time later, after this **lucid interval**, the patient may start to develop localising signs of raised intracranial pressure, with weakness on the side opposite to the lesion and a fixed dilated pupil on the side of the lesion.

Rapid recognition of the possibility of an extradural haemorrhage should result in immediate imaging using a CT scan or MRI, followed by surgical decompression using burr holes, followed by raising a flap. The moment that the pressure is relieved the patient miraculously recovers.

Brain injury

Direct damage to the brain itself will be made worse by bleeding and swelling secondary to the trauma of the injury. Controlled dehydration, hyperventilation reducing blood carbon dioxide and high-dose steroids are all used to try to minimise the secondary damage caused by the brain swelling inside a rigid container (the skull), but so far there is no conclusive evidence that any of these techniques improve the outcome. However, what does make a difference is making sure that the brain is well perfused and well oxygenated.

Chronic subdural haemorrhage

In the elderly a trivial fall can lead to a small subdural haemorrhage that may continue to expand long after the original trauma has been forgotten. The patient may show a gradual deterioration in mental faculties over a period of weeks or even months. The underlying cause will only be revealed once a scan has been performed.

Raised intracranial pressure

In the acute phase of raised intracranial pressure, the patient's conscious state will be depressed and respiration will be reduced, as will the pulse, although paradoxically blood pressure may go up (the opposite of hypovolaemic shock). If pressure continues to rise, the patient's conscious state will deteriorate and they will become rigid and spastic (**decerebrate**). Eventually the brainstem will be driven down into the foramen magnum, leading to coning and death.

Rehabilitation

Although the central nervous system is thought to have very limited powers of regeneration, the brain does seem to be able to achieve some recovery by **plasticity** – recruiting new pathways to perform tasks where the old pathway has been damaged. This appears to occur much more easily in the young than in the old, but either way occurs over a period of many months. During that time the patient will need considerable social and physical support, as their personality can be profoundly altered and their behaviour become very disruptive.

Tips

- In head injuries check and recheck ABC, intubating if necessary
- Check for other injuries
- Remember hypoglycaemia and drugs. Coma may have caused the accident, rather than the accident causing concussion
- A lucid interval followed by deterioration may indicate an extradural emergency

40 Fractures and dislocations

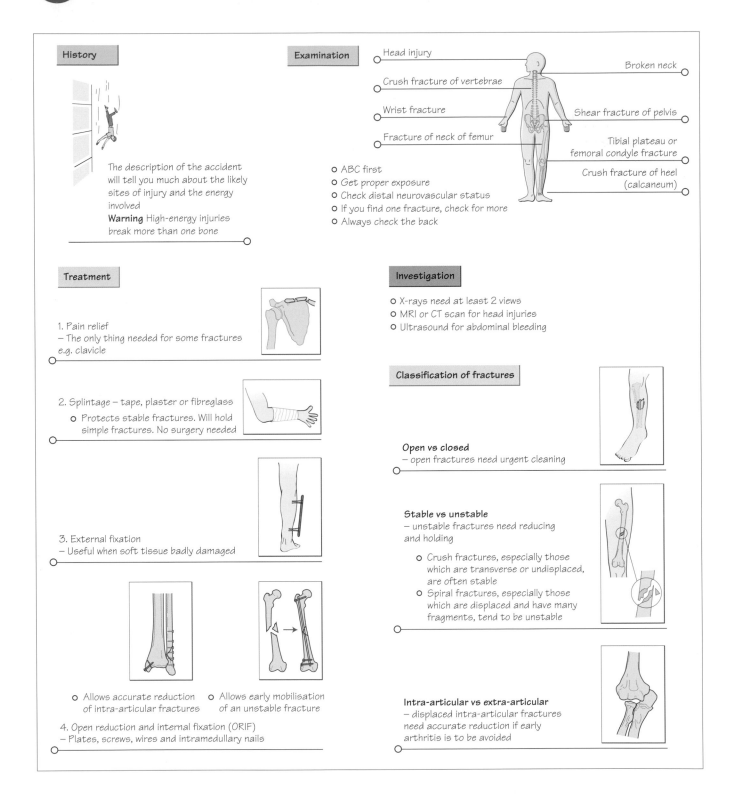

History

The description of the accident will tell you much about the likely sites of injury and the energy involved
Warning High-energy injuries break more than one bone

Examination

- Head injury
- Crush fracture of vertebrae
- Wrist fracture
- Fracture of neck of femur
- Broken neck
- Shear fracture of pelvis
- Tibial plateau or femoral condyle fracture
- Crush fracture of heel (calcaneum)

- ABC first
- Get proper exposure
- Check distal neurovascular status
- If you find one fracture, check for more
- Always check the back

Treatment

1. Pain relief
   – The only thing needed for some fractures e.g. clavicle

2. Splintage – tape, plaster or fibreglass
   - Protects stable fractures. Will hold simple fractures. No surgery needed

3. External fixation
   – Useful when soft tissue badly damaged

- Allows accurate reduction of intra-articular fractures
- Allows early mobilisation of an unstable fracture

4. Open reduction and internal fixation (ORIF)
   – Plates, screws, wires and intramedullary nails

Investigation

- X-rays need at least 2 views
- MRI or CT scan for head injuries
- Ultrasound for abdominal bleeding

Classification of fractures

Open vs closed
– open fractures need urgent cleaning

Stable vs unstable
– unstable fractures need reducing and holding

- Crush fractures, especially those which are transverse or undisplaced, are often stable
- Spiral fractures, especially those which are displaced and have many fragments, tend to be unstable

Intra-articular vs extra-articular
– displaced intra-articular fractures need accurate reduction if early arthritis is to be avoided

Causes

If the load going through a limb exceeds its strength then either the bone will break or the capsule around a joint will tear and the joint surfaces will come apart partially (**subluxation**) or totally (**dislocation**).

A normal force can be adequate to break a bone if it is in a direction to which the bone or joint has little resistance (e.g. a spiral fracture of the humerus in arm wrestlers). It can also occur if the bone has been weakened by disease. Patients with severe osteoporosis may fall having sustained a fracture of the neck of the femur simply when walking. The fall does not cause the fracture, the fracture leads to the fall.

Repeated loads can also damage the bone by fatiguing the mineral crystals. Long-distance runners may sustain a spontaneous break in the tibia in this way – a **stress fracture**.

Shape and direction of injury

1 Shape of the fracture. This is determined by the direction of force applied:

- Spiral fractures result from twisting.
- Crush fractures result from excess longitudinal load.
- Transverse fractures result from bending forces.
- Very high impact energies tend to explode bones into multiple fragments.

2 Direction of the dislocation. A joint is more susceptible to dislocation if the patient has lax ligaments or if there is damage to the capsule from a previous dislocation. The direction of the dislocation is again dependent on the direction of force applied.

History

A fracture or dislocation is usually quite easy to diagnose. The patient will be able to describe what they have felt or heard. A dislocation may then have relocated so this history is important.

Examination

Do not forget to check distal neurovascular status, then use the 'look, feel, move' system to check for:

- wounds on the skin;
- bleeding into the soft tissues;
- deformity of bones and joints.

Movement needs to be performed carefully, watching the patient's face, testing for ruptures of muscles and ligaments, instability of joints and even crepitus in bones.

Investigation

At least two X-rays will be needed centred on the site of injury, aligned at right angles to each other.

Classification of fractures

1 Stable versus unstable. Some fractures (especially those involving a simple crush) are stable. This means that they will not move unless considerable force is applied. In other cases fractures are unstable, especially spiral or comminuted (multi-fragmentary) fractures.

2 Open versus closed. A wound close to a fractured bone converts the fracture from a closed one to an open one. Open fractures are contaminated until otherwise proven. If the wound is not cleaned out at once, then infection will set in. Once infection has established itself in the bone, then it is said that it can never be eradicated – it may always break out again. It is better to prevent **osteomyelitis** than try to cure it.

3 Viable versus avascular. If a bone fragment loses its blood supply as a result of the fracture or the stripping of soft tissues then that fragment may not be able to acquire a blood supply quickly enough to heal and so may die and need removing or replacing.

4 Intra-articular versus extra-articular. Fractures extending into a joint surface present special problems. If they are not reduced exactly (less than a 2 mm step in the articular surface) then **early arthritis** in that joint is inevitable. The bone fragments are also more likely to have lost their blood supply, so healing may be a problem.

Growth plate fractures in children

Fractures across the growth plates of children's bones can interfere with the ability of that bone to grow and need handling with special care. Every effort must be made to prevent the epiphyseal plate from producing a deformity.

Management

The management of a fracture or dislocation usually involves reduction and then holding.

1 Reduction. In order to reduce a fracture it is useful to understand the direction of the force that created it. Paradoxically, the first move is to increase the deformity in the direction of the original damaging force. This allows the joint or fracture fragments to be separated from each other without damaging the capsule or periosteum, which is intact on the inside of the deformity. This is then used as the hinge and the guide to bring the structures back into their correct relationship.

2 Fixation. Once reduced the fracture or dislocation needs to be held to prevent it displacing again.

- Sometimes a simple sling will be adequate.
- In other cases bone fragments may need to be held exactly in position with a plate and screws.
- Plaster of Paris is cheap and simple to use but does not hold fractures very precisely and is a great inconvenience to the patient while they wait for the fracture to heal. However, this method may be ideal for fractures in children, which heal quickly and remodel as they grow.
- In patients with fractures through metastases, quick and strong fixation with an intramedullary nail will allow them to get home as quickly as possible.

Complications

Fractures can unite in a bad position (**malunion**) or heal slowly or even not at all (**non-union**). Failure to unite can be a result of poor blood supply. In this case the bone ends just wither away. A little movement stimulates bone healing. Too much movement produces exuberant new bone, but a failure to bridge the cleft. Bone grafting and secure fixation of the fracture may be needed to treat delayed union or non-union.

Stiffness and weakness can be a problem after fractures or dislocations. Physiotherapy has a key role in rehabilitation to full function.

Osteotomies

Bones can be broken deliberately to correct deformity or even to lengthen limbs. External fixator frames can then be used to move fragments of bone, providing the speed is not so high that non-union results or too slow so that the osteotomy unites before adequate movement has been achieved.

Tips

- Check ABC first, then for other injuries, before focusing on the presenting injury
- Check distal neurovascular status
- Open fractures need cleaning out to prevent osteomyelitis
- Fractures into joints need exact reduction
- Fractures into the growth plates of children's bones need special care
- Pathological fractures in the elderly need quick fixation to return their mobility

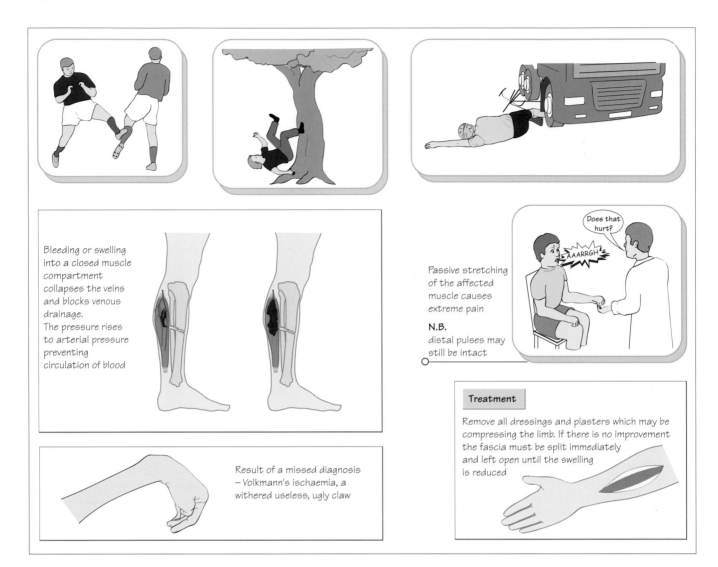

Bleeding or swelling into a closed muscle compartment collapses the veins and blocks venous drainage.
The pressure rises to arterial pressure preventing circulation of blood

Passive stretching of the affected muscle causes extreme pain

N.B.
distal pulses may still be intact

Does that hurt?

AAARRGH

Result of a missed diagnosis – Volkmann's ischaemia, a withered useless, ugly claw

Treatment

Remove all dressings and plasters which may be compressing the limb. If there is no improvement the fascia must be split immediately and left open until the swelling is reduced

Pathophysiology

If there has been damage to the blood supply of a limb or severe damage to the soft tissues (with or without a fracture), then there may be swelling or haemorrhage of the muscles. Some muscles are enclosed in a rigid fascia. If they swell, the pressure inside that compartment may rise and actually cut off the blood supply to the muscle. Over a period of hours the muscle dies, and is then replaced by fibrous tissue that contracts. The end result is a **Volkmann's ischaemic contracture** – a useless, withered, clawed limb. Even those muscles that are not in a fixed fascia can behave in the same way if the limb is encased in a tight dressing or a closed plaster. Ischaemia can therefore be iatrogenic (caused by a doctor), and all dressings and casts should be split if there is any possibility that the limb might continue to swell.

Diagnosis

Compartment syndrome is diagnosed by having a 'high index of suspicion'. There are said to be five Ps – **pain**, **paralysis**, **pallor**,

paraesthesia and **pulseless** – but these are also present in the ischaemic limb. Not all of these need to be present for a compartment syndrome to be diagnosed. Only pain and paralysis are reliable features. The pulse can still be present as the artery passing through the compartment has stiff walls that may resist the pressure even when the tissues in the compartment are not being perfused.

Late or chronic compartment syndrome is rare, so if late pain is a problem, consider **deep infection** (especially gangrene) and **regional pain syndrome** (sometime called Sudek's atrophy or reflex sympathetic dystrophy).

Presentation

The commonest presentation is being called to see a patient (especially a child) in whom there has been trauma and who is now complaining of severe and increasing pain just at a time when the pain should be settling down. This could be after an elective operation but is usually after trauma. It can be difficult to distinguish between a patient who is anxious and a developing compartment syndrome. It is best to be on the safe side and act on the assumption that it is a compartment syndrome.

Examination

A reliable physical sign is to distract the patient and then flex and extend the digits at the end of the limb in question. If the patient cries out in pain (because the ischaemic muscles are being stretched) then the diagnosis has been made.

Treatment

The treatment of a compartment syndrome is a surgical emergency.

• The first thing to do is to divide the plaster and dressings in case it is these that are constricting the circulation.

• If there is not an immediate improvement, the patient must go to the operating theatre and the compartments in question should be opened up from end to end.

If there is no compartment syndrome found, then no great harm has been done, and the wound can be closed the following day. If there is a compartment syndrome the muscle will pout out and if it has been caught early enough the muscle will reperfuse. If it has been left too late and it is literally a matter of a few hours then the muscle will be dead and will need excising. Either way the wound should be left open initially, then a second look taken a day later when it will be clear what is the likely outcome, and the swelling will have gone down.

Tips

• Always split a dressing or plaster on a limb which may still swell
• Have a high index of suspicion for compartment syndrome
• If stretching the affected muscles causes pain, take action at once
• First remove all casts and dressings in case they are the cause
• Urgent fasciotomy is needed if there is not immediate improvement

Self-assessment case studies: questions

Case 1: Acute joint disease

A 42-year-old man presents to casualty with a painful and swollen right knee, which he attributes to an old football injury 'flaring up again'. He is otherwise well but is unable to bear weight. His medical past includes insulin-dependent diabetes and psoriasis. He is a businessman and drinks 32 units of alcohol per week.

1 *What elements of the history so far are helpful in forming a differential diagnosis and why?*

Further questioning reveals a history of a red eye.

2 *What other rheumatological diagnoses might link this symptom with his arthropathy and what other features would you ask about to confirm or refute these possibilities?*

The red eye transpires to be a history of subconjunctival haemorrhage and unrelated to his current presentation.

3 *What is your first-line investigation in this patient and why?*

A diagnosis of acute gout is made.

4 *How would you treat this patient? And if he suffered recurrent attacks?*

Case 2: Initial management of polytrauma

A 19-year-old motorcyclist had just bought a 1000 cc super motorcycle. While negotiating a corner, it appears that he lost control and the bike skidded into the path of an oncoming 4×4. The rider's body hit the vertical front of the vehicle obliquely bouncing across into the ditch. The car driver was uninjured and used a mobile phone to summon assistance. A paramedic was on site within 10 minutes. The helmet was removed and the rider was put onto a spineboard and brought in blue and unresponsive arriving 25 minutes after the 999 call.

1 *Describe your initial management.*

As soon as the leathers and clothing were cut away, it became clear that the left femur was sticking out through the skin of the mid-thigh.

2 *What must now be checked?*

3 *What are the principles of treatment of the broken femur?*

4 *What options are available for fixing the fracture?*

Case 3: Rheumatoid arthritis

A 28-year-old woman is referred to the clinic with painful hands. Her symptoms began several months ago and now all of her metacarpophalangeals are affected. Her fingers are stiff for several hours each morning and swollen for most of the day.

1 *Does she meet all the ACR (American College of Rheumatology) diagnostic criteria for rheumatoid arthritis?*

2 *What role would measurement of rheumatoid factor play in this patient?*

The patient is diagnosed with rheumatoid arthritis and commenced on methotrexate as first-line disease-modifying therapy.

3 *What information does she need to be given concerning this treatment?*

Several months later she presents as an emergency with increasing shortness of breath.

4 *What is your differential diagnosis and how would you investigate her further?*

After several years of DMARD (disease-modifying antirheumatic drug) therapy her disease remains uncontrolled. Examination reveals classic bony deformities and muscle wasting in her hands.

5 *List the causes of small muscle wasting in patients with rheumatoid arthritis.*

The patient has read about TNF (tumour necrosis factor) blockade on the internet and is keen to try it.

6 *What are the current guidelines for use of TNF blockade in patients with rheumatoid arthritis?*

Case 4: Septic arthritis

A 4-year-old child is brought in by her mother. For 2 days she has been off colour, and is now toxic and generally unwell. The child is crying, wants to be picked up by her mother but screams when her mother tries. There appears to be extreme pain in the left leg and she will not take any weight through that leg. It is difficult to localise the source of the pain – it could be the knee, the hip or even referred from the back.

1 *What would you look for on examination?*

2 *What investigations would you do to confirm/exclude the diagnosis?*

3 *What is the treatment?*

Case 5: Limps in the elderly

A 75-year-old presents with increasing pain in the right leg on walking. He also describes stiffness in the left hip, and mentions that the leg now feels shorter than the other side.

1 *What is the likely diagnosis?*

2 *What questions might you ask to determine the severity of symptoms?*

3 *What four classic features of this condition might you see on X-ray?*

4 *List four treatment options.*

Case 6: Osteoporosis

A 72-year-old woman is admitted to Accident and Emergency following a fall. The medical team are concerned that she may have sustained low trauma fractures due to osteoporosis.

1 *What are the commonest sites for osteoporotic fracture?*

2 *List the risk factors for osteoporosis that you would seek in the history.*

3 *How would you confirm the diagnosis of osteoporosis?*

4 *What is the first-line treatment for the primary prevention of osteoporosis in this patient? What instructions would you give her on how and when to take this therapy?*

Case 7: Problems in the hand

A 60-year-old labourer who works with pneumatic drills and erects scaffolding presents with an inability to straighten his little and ring fingers of his dominant hand. It has been coming on for some time. He says his father developed the same problem at the same age. He smokes 20 a day and is a hard drinker too.

1 *What is the diagnosis?*
2 *What is the likely natural history if this is left untreated?*
3 *What four features in the history given predispose him to this condition?*
4 *What is the surgical treatment and postoperative care?*

Case 8: More problems in the hand

A 45-year-old woman starts noticing that she is becoming increasingly clumsy. She also notices that the index and middle finger of her right dominant hand go numb at night. If she hangs her hand out of bed and shakes it, the symptoms are relieved.

1 *What is the likely diagnosis?*
2 *What might you notice on examination?*
3 *What investigation might you use to confirm/exclude the diagnosis?*
4 *What is the surgical treatment?*

Case 9: Systemic lupus erythematosis

A 24-year-old patient presents with arthropathy and a rash. Her ANA (antinuclear antibody) is positive (1/640) and you are concerned that she has developed systemic lupus erythematosus (SLE).

1 *What types of rash are associated with SLE?*
2 *What questions would you ask in the history to confirm the diagnosis of SLE?*

The patient meets the diagnostic criteria for lupus. Her immunology reveals positive dsDNA, Ro and La; lupus anticoagulant is also detected.

3 *What other symptoms may this patient experience? And if she were pregnant?*

At a routine clinic visit she complains of swollen ankles. Her blood pressure is elevated and a urine dipstick is positive for protein and blood.

4 *How would you proceed?*

Case 10: Complications of fractures

An 8-year-old child falls from a tree landing on her outstretched arm. She was not knocked out, but complains of pain in the right arm. The right elbow is deformed.

1 *What is the likely fracture?*
2 *What must be checked in that arm?*

You reduce the fracture, and put the arm into a back-slab plaster with the elbow flexed to hold the fracture reduced. The child is admitted to hospital for observation. Late that night you are called by the nurse to see the child, because the child is in severe pain despite analgesia, and will not settle. The sensation and circulation to the fingers is OK.

3 *What is the dangerous diagnosis that must now be excluded?*
4 *What simple examination/test can you perform that confirms the diagnosis?*
5 *Describe what you would do first to try to relieve the symptoms, and what you would have to do then if the symptoms did not resolve.*

Case 11: Congenital abnormalities

A child is born full-term following a breech delivery with one foot bent downwards and inwards. This is the mother's first child, and the pregnancy was uncomplicated.

1 *What is the likely diagnosis?*
2 *List two causes and/or associations with this condition.*
3 *What are the treatment options?*

Self-assessment case studies: answers

Case 1: Acute joint disease

1 The most crucial piece of information is that the patient is well. The diagnosis to rule out in every case is septic arthritis, and this seems unlikely in this scenario. However, his diabetes is a risk factor for infection, and a careful history of the previous injury might reveal a route of entry for bacteria. Although sports injuries can cause recurrent problems, acute flares of swelling and pain are unusual in the absence of a clear precipitating event. His psoriasis may indicate the development of a large-joint psoriatic arthropathy, but psoriasis is also a risk factor for gout, and his alcohol intake would certainly put him at risk of this.

2 The combination of a painful red eye and arthropathy raises the possibility of anterior uveitis or scleritis in association with one of the following:
- Reiter's syndrome (check for a history of urethritis or gastrointestinal upset, circinate balanitis, keratoderma blennorrhagia).
- Enteropathic arthropathy (history of abdominal pain or bloody diarrhoea, erythema nodosum).
- Ankylosing spondylitis (inflammatory back pain).

3 Joint fluid aspiration to rule out septic arthritis and to diagnose gout.

4 First-line treatment for gout is a non-steroidal anti-inflammatory (NSAID). If he continues to experience attacks, a urate-lowering therapy such as allopurinol should be considered. All patients with gout should attempt lifestyle modification. In this instance, a reduction in his alcohol intake is crucial. Additional risk factors in his diet would also need to be addressed.

See Chapter 24 for further details.

Case 2: Initial management of polytrauma

1 ABC:
- A. Check airway with cervical spine control.
- B. Breathing: give 100% oxygen at 15 l/min; check for pneumothorax.
- C. Circulation: introduce two wide-bore cannulae. Take bloods for cross-match, haemoglobin, glucose, urea and electrolytes, and drug screen.

2 Distal neurovascular status.

3 The fracture is open and potentially contaminated. The wound must therefore be opened and cleaned. All contaminating material should be washed out, and dead tissue excised. If it is not possible to be sure that the wound is clean, then it should not be closed. The wound should be packed and then inspected daily until it is clean. The fracture needs to be reduced, and then held. The operation should be covered by prophylactic antibiotics. The patient should be mobilised as soon as practicable.

4 Options include intramedullary nail with locking screws; plate and screws; external fixator (Ilizarov or conventional); balanced traction; plaster or brace. An intramedullary nail allows secure fixation and early mobilisation but infection is a dangerous complication. A plate with screws needs a much longer incision, but will also give secure fixation. An external fixator is very difficult to apply, especially in the thigh where the soft tissues are deep so the pins rub on the muscle. Traction is safe but takes many weeks with the patient languishing in a hospital bed. A plaster or brace would be almost impossible to fit to a thigh so that the fracture could be held.

See Chapters 34 and 40 for further details.

Case 3: Rheumatoid arthritis

1 No, but enough to make the diagnosis! The diagnostic criteria stipulate at least four of the following:
- Morning stiffness: duration > 1 hour (for > 6 weeks).
- Arthritis of at least three joints: soft tissue swelling (for > 6 weeks).
- Arthritis of hand joints: MCPs, PIPs or wrist (for > 6 weeks).
- Symmetrical arthritis: at least one area (for > 6 weeks).
- Rheumatoid nodules.
- Positive rheumatoid factor.
- Radiographic changes: periarticular erosions.

2 Rhematoid factor positivity is associated with more severe disease and a higher incidence of extra-articular manifestations.

3 Methotrexate is effective and generally well tolerated. Side effects include nausea and oral ulcers. Regular blood tests are used to screen for myelosuppression and hepatitis. An idiosyncratic (and reversible) allergic alveolitis/pneumonitis can occur and pre-treatment lung function testing and chest X-ray is advised. Pregnancy is contraindicated as methotrexate is a folic acid antagonist.

4 Differential diagnoses:
- Respiratory disease:
  Pleural effusion
  Pulmonary fibrosis
  Allergic alveolitis due to methotrexate therapy
  Bronchiolitis obliterans (rare)
  Cryptogenic organising pneumonia (rare).

Investigations include arterial blood gases, chest X-ray and lung function testing.
- Symptomatic anaemia:
  Anaemia of chronic disease
  Gastrointestinal blood loss due to NSAID use
  Myelosuppression due to methotrexate therapy
  Associated B12 deficiency (pernicious anaemia).

Investigations include haematinics and endoscopy.

5 Causes include:
- Disuse atrophy.
- Compression neuropathy (median and/or ulnar).
- Cervical myelopathy.
- Mononeuritis multiplex due to rheumatoid vasculitis.

6 NICE (National Institute for Clinical Excellence) has stipulated that patients must have active disease and have failed two or more DMARDs (disease modifying anti-rheumatic drugs), of which one must be methotrexate. All patients must be screened for TB prior to commencing therapy.

See Chapter 22 for further details.

Case 4: Septic arthritis

1 Pyrexia, redness, swelling and pain on moving the affected joint.
2 Ultrasound. If effusion is found, aspirate and send for microscopy, culture and sensitivity.
3 High-dose intravenous antibiotics. Open drainage if no immediate settling.

See Chapters 16, 25 and 30 for further details.

Case 5: Limps in the elderly

1 Osteoarthritic hip.
2 Ask about pain-waking at night, regular painkillers and walking aids. Is there difficulty with getting socks and shoes on, and getting in and out of the bath?
3 Loss of joint space, osteophyte formation, subchondral sclerosis and cysts in the bone below the joint.
4 Painkillers, physiotherapy, home aids and joint replacement.

See Chapters 15, 17 and 33 for further details.

Case 6: Osteoporosis

1 Vertebral body, neck of femur and distal radius.
2 Factors include:
   • Maternal family history of hip fracture.
   • Oestrogen deficiency.
   • Corticosteroid therapy.
   • Low body mass index ($< 19\,kg/m^2$).
   • Smoking and excess alcohol.
   • Anorexia nervosa (low weight, menstrual irregularity, low calcium intake).
   • Endocrine syndromes (hyperparathyroidism, hyperthyroidism, Cushing's syndrome).
   • Inflammatory arthropathy (probably due to increased IL-1 and TNFα levels).
   • Prolonged immobilisation.
3 Osteoporosis is diagnosed using a dual energy X-ray absorptiometry (DEXA) scan. This allows a measurement of the bone mineral density (BMD) at the lumbar spine and proximal femur for comparison with that of the young normal mean. The T score in osteoporosis is > 2.5 SD below the young normal mean (i.e. T > –2.5).
4 Bisphosphonate and vitamin D/calcium supplementation is the treatment of choice. In order to improve its poor bioavailability, and reduce gastrointestinal side effects, patients must take their bisphosphonate on an empty stomach, with plenty of water, remain upright for 30 minutes after ingestion and have nothing to eat or drink for a further 30 minutes.

See Chapter 26 for further details.

Case 7: Problems in the hand

1 Dupuytren's contracture.
2 Steady progression to fixed contracture.
3 Alcohol intake, liver disorder, family history and prolonged use of vibrating equipment.
4 Excise the palmar fascia, then physiotherapy to regain mobility.

See Chapters 7 and 34 for further details.

Case 8: More problems in the hand

1 Carpal tunnel syndrome.
2 Wasting of the thenar eminence and weakness of opposition.
3 Nerve conduction studies.
4 Decompression of the carpal tunnel roof.

See Chapters 6 and 7 for further details.

Case 9: Systemic lupus erythematosis

1 Malar rash, discoid rash and photosensitivity.
2 Ask about the following;
   • Details of the rash (distribution, scars, exacerbations, etc.).
   • History of the arthropathy (features of early morning stiffness?).
   • History of oral ulcers?
   • Previous episodes of serositis – pericarditis or pleurisy?
   • Remember that symptoms such as Raynaud's phenomenon and fatigue, although common in lupus, do not contribute to the diagnostic criteria.
3 dsDNA has a high specificity for SLE and levels may fluctuate with disease activity. The Ro and La antibodies suggest a Sjögren's syndrome pattern of disease, i.e. dry eyes, dry mouth and vaginal dryness. Fatigue is a particular problem in these patients. Lupus anticoagulant puts her at risk of thromboembolic phenomenon. In the pregnant lupus patient with this Ro/La positivity, neonatal lupus and fetal heart block are a concern; those with lupus anticoagulant are at risk of deep venous thrombosis and/or miscarriage.
4 The patient may have developed renal lupus. The urine should be sent for microscopy to examine for the presence of red cell casts – evidence of glomerular bleeding in glomerulonephritis. A 24-hour collection of urine should be undertaken to quantify the proteinuria. The case must then be discussed with renal physicians for consideration of a renal biopsy. If glomerulonephritis is confirmed, aggressive immunosuppression should be instituted. Meticulous blood pressure control is mandatory.

See Chapter 27 for further details.

Case 10: Complications of fractures

1 Supracondylar fracture of the humerus.
2 Distal neurovascular status.
3 Compartment syndrome.
4 Pain on passive stretching of the muscles – stretch the fingers.
5 Split the plaster, then fasciotomy if there is not a resolution of symptoms.

See Chapters 5, 8 and 41 for further details.

Case 11: Congenital abnormalities

1 Club foot (talipes equinovarus).

2 Oligohydramnios. Other congenital abnormalities such as spina bifida and congenital dislocation of the hip are associated with this condition. Position in uterus.

3 If the deformity is only a result of bad positioning in the uterus, then serial strapping of the foot can gradually correct the deformity. However, if the deformity is a developmental defect then surgical release of the tight structures will be needed if the foot is to grow as normally as possible.

See Chapter 30 for further details.

Index

at a Glance

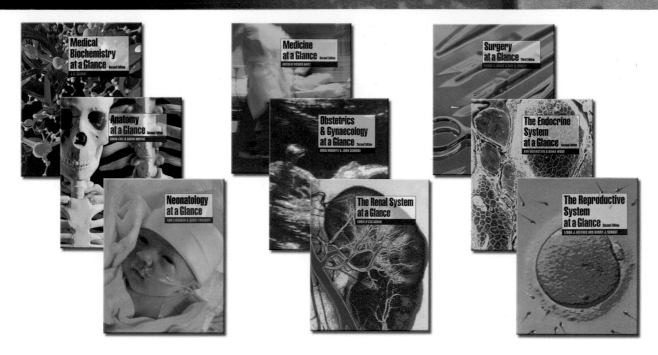

- The most simple and concise approach to all your subjects
  - Each bite-sized chapter covered in a double-page spread with key facts and fundamentals and a summary diagram
    - Perfect for exam preparation and use on clinical rotations

Titles in the at a Glance series

- Anatomy at a Glance
- The Cardiovascular System at a Glance
- Critical Care Medicine at a Glance
- The Endocrine System at a Glance
- The Gastrointestinal System at a Glance
- Haematology at a Glance
- History and Examination at a Glance
- Immunology at a Glance
- Medical Biochemistry at a Glance
- Medical Genetics at a Glance
- Medical Microbiology and Infection at a Glance
- Medical Pharmacology at a Glance
- Medical Statistics at a Glance

- Medicine at a Glance
- Metabolism at a Glance
- Neonatology at a Glance
- Neuroscience at a Glance
- Obstetrics and Gynaecology at a Glance
- Ophthalmology at a Glance
- Paediatrics at a Glance
- Physiology at a Glance
- Psychiatry at a Glance
- The Renal System at a Glance
- The Reproductive System at a Glance
- The Respiratory System at a Glance
- Surgery at a Glance

www.blackwellmedstudent.com

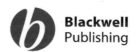

Blackwell Publishing

LECTURE NOTES

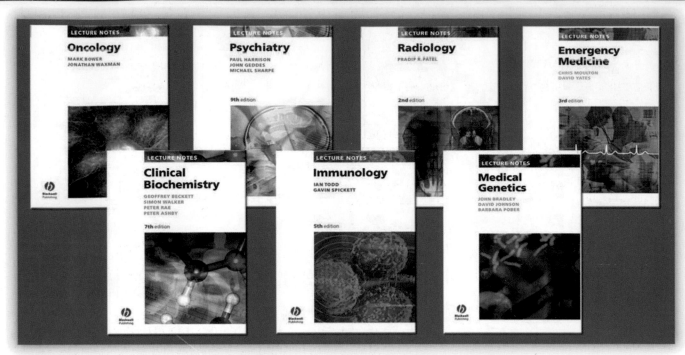

- Concise learning guides for all your subjects
- Focused on what you need to know
- Tried and Trusted

Titles in the LECTURE NOTES series

- Cardiology
- Clinical Anaesthesia
- Clinical Biochemistry
- Clinical Medicine
- Clinical Pharmacology and Therapeutics
- Clinical Skills
- Dermatology
- Diseases of the Ear, Nose and Throat
- Emergency Medicine
- Epidemiology and Public Health Medicine
- General Surgery
- Geriatric Medicine
- Haematology
- Human Physiology
- Immunology
- Infectious Diseases
- Medical Genetics
- Medical Law and Ethics
- Medical Microbiology and Infection
- Neurology
- Obstetrics and Gynaecology
- Oncology
- Ophthalmology
- Orthopaedics and Fractures
- Paediatrics
- Psychiatry
- Radiology
- Respiratory Medicine
- Tropical Medicine
- Urology

www.blackwellmedstudent.com 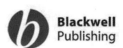 Blackwell Publishing